P9-CJX-048

WINNING THE ENDGAME

WINNING THE ENDGAME

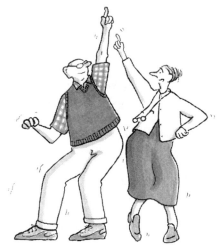

A Guide to Aging Wisely and Dying Well

BY RAY BROWN

ILLUSTRATIONS BY JULIA SUITS

Text copyright © 2016 by Ray Brown.
Illustrations copyright © 2016 by Julia Suits.
All rights reserved. No part of this book may
be reproduced in any form without written
permission from the publisher.

978-0-9980628-0-8 paperback
978-0-9980628-1-5 ebook

Manufactured in the United States of America.

Produced by Jay Schaefer Books, San Francisco.
Designed by Pamela Geismar, Domino Design.
Typeset by Jessica Dacher, Dacher Designery.

FOR ANNIE B, LOVE OF MY LIFE.

CONTENTS

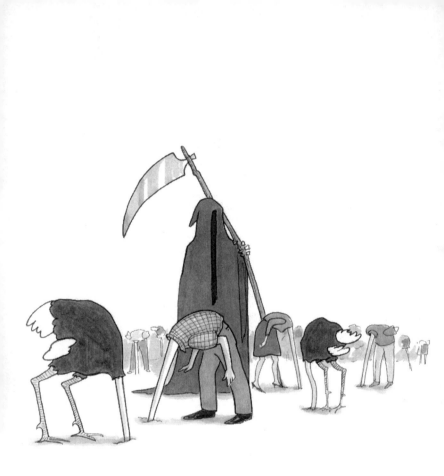

INTRODUCTION

Age happens. If you're lucky.

America is a nation of death ostriches. They're desperately trying to hide from the dude in the black hoodie holding a razor-sharp scythe. Death ostriches hope if they stick their heads deeply enough into the sands of oblivion and stand *really* still, then maybe—just maybe—Death won't find them.

Fat chance. By misdirecting their energy into denial of mortality, death ostriches reduce the odds of achieving a good death. That's a dumb trade.

Death always wins at hide-and-seek. But, if you play the endgame well, Death may grant you a peaceful pass at home surrounded by your loved ones. In my book, that's a win.

Winning the Endgame will help optimize the rest of your life. If your idea of happiness is living as well as possible for as long as possible and then slipping gently into the next great adventure, *Winning the Endgame* is the yellow brick road to your personal Oz.

Here's what you'll discover along the way:

Part I—Aging Wisely

Chapter 1: Staying Power. Is 70 the new 50? What are your odds of living to 100? (It could happen.) Here you'll find out if you've meandered past middle age and delve into how much longer you're likely to live. That neatly segues into staying power, your ability to outlast adversity.

Chapter 2: Financing Ideas for Homeowners. This chapter is full of fascinating financial considerations for homeowners who don't plan to sell their dream house. It red flags a devastating mistake many homeowners make shortly before they retire. If you're a renter, you have 100 percent guilt-free permission to skip to Chapter 4.

Chapter 3: Selling Your House. We consider the pros and cons of *rightsizing*—not downsizing—your house. You'll see the relationship you have with your house for what it really is—unrequited love.

Chapter 4: Endgame Housing Alternatives. Shelter strategies for everyone. Why? Because you gotta live somewhere.

Chapter 5: Risk Management. As your staying power diminishes, you become increasingly vulnerable. You can't eliminate risk, but you can manage it to enhance your odds of a happy ending. Use these strategies to defend against the Fearsome Four Risks.

Part II—Dying Well

Chapter 6: Advance Directive. Preparing to exit gracefully requires long-term planning skill and the courage to confront death without blinking. I'll guide you through a living will and a durable health care power of attorney, the components of an Advance Directive (AD). You'll see how to use your AD to begin tough-love conversations with family and friends who someday may have to make difficult decisions on your behalf.

Chapter 7: A Good Death. As Kenny Rogers said in *The Gambler*, "Ya gotta know when to hold 'em, know when to fold 'em." We delve into palliative care, hospice, and dying with dignity.

You won't say "TL; DR" ("Too Long; Didn't Read") about *Winning the Endgame* (henceforth *"WTEG"*). It's concise. You'll probably finish *WTEG* in a couple of hours. It isn't filled with endless stacks of statistics that have the life span of fruit flies. Wherever possible, I connect statistical dots to form conclusions you can use to reimagine your life.

WTEG brings death out of the closet. Note that I just used the D word again. Go ahead. Say it with me—"death, death, death, death." See. Nothing bad happens.

If you think *WTEG* is a downer, you're dead wrong. I'm not saying you'll laugh your head off (an awkward way to go), but you will be pleasantly surprised. *WTEG* is cheerful, not morbid—*Harold and Maude*, not *Hamlet.* I'm Paul Revere, not Dr. Kevorkian.

You're equally off base to figure that you don't need *WTEG* because you're as healthy as the proverbial ox. "Healthy" is a word used to describe the slowest rate of dying. No matter how *healthy* you are now, you're gonna die. Life is 100 percent fatal. If this comes as a shock, you're too young to read *WTEG*. Put it away till you're mature enough to calmly contemplate your endgame.

If, however, the thought of a tombstone with your name carved on it doesn't freak you out, congrats. You passed my first test. There will be others.

The endgame begins on your 60th birthday and concludes when you toddle off to the big sleep. Whether your finale is grand or tragic depends upon how you position yourself now. Winning the endgame requires *relentlessly ruthless realism*. Throw away your rose-colored glasses. Embrace the world as it is, not as you wish it were.

You don't need *WTEG* if you're absolutely, unequivocally certain you'll spend the rest of your life in perfect health with nary a natural disaster, drunk driver, fractured hip, or ruinous recession to mess up your idyllic existence. If you're nimble enough to dodge the muck that life flings at ordinary mortals, know that I envy you.

However, if cascades of uncertainty drench you daily, welcome to my world. *WTEG* will help you make worst-case-scenario contingency plans. There'd be no need for contingency plans in a perfect world. As a realist, you know sewage happens whether you're prepared or not. When it comes to dying, I admire Woody Allen. He's not afraid of dying. Woody just doesn't want to be there when it happens. My feelings exactly.

As a student of death, I avidly read the In Memory section of paid death notices in my newspaper. Every morning I scan the fresh harvest of prom pix, high school graduation head shots, faded wedding photos, and blurry WWII snapshots. Then I read the glowing tributes to the newly departed. Decades of study have taught me two things:

The second worst death notice starts, "After a courageous [funeral director lingo for suffered stoically] battle with [fill in the blank with a nasty way to kick the bucket, such as ALS, lung cancer, or getting gnawed to death by beavers] . . ."

The worst death notice begins, "After a long, courageous battle with . . ."

Have you noticed that lately more and more people don't seem to get your references? I'm keenly aware of this problem. For example, in the brief time we've known each other, I've referred to Paul Revere, Dr. Kevorkian, *Harold and Maude, Hamlet,* the yellow brick road, Oz, Woody Allen, prom photos, and World War II. I hope you got my drift.

Inadvertent obscurity first bludgeoned me in 2006 when I was managing a residential real estate company. Bill, our newest agent, came into my office one evening utterly dejected. He overheard a couple of experienced agents say he wouldn't make it selling homes because he was too young and had no contacts.

I told Bill not to worry; that I wouldn't have hired him if I didn't think he had the right stuff. Bill remained steadfastly glum.

"OK," I finally said. "You're not talking to Ray Brown anymore. I'm Harry Truman. The buck stops here. What do you want me to do?"

"Who's Harry Truman?" he replied.

When I told a pal about this at lunch the next day his response was, "Bullshit, Ray. Nobody's that dumb."

"Do you know who Harry Truman is?" I asked our 20-something waitress when she brought our burgers.

"The name's familiar."

I said there'd be more tests. This chapter is a screening tool. If you think my references are incomprehensible, don't finish *WTEG*. It's for the silver tsunami of baby boomers born between 1946 and 1964. If you're a mite older, don't sweat it. I hark back to 1939.

If you're a boomer, we have much in common. Like me, you've actually touched ancient relics such as 78-, 33⅓-, and 45-rpm records; rotary dial telephones; fountain pens; manual typewriters and carbon paper. Today they're as obsolete as telegrams and "Be kind. Rewind." (Another obscure reference.)

Presidents used to be old guys. The first election I voted in pitted Richard Nixon against John F. Kennedy, both elderly from my perspective of 21 years. The last time I was younger than the president, George H. W. Bush (b. 1924) was in the White House. Today's college-age kids have only known boomer presidents—Clinton (b. 1946), Bush II (b. 1946), and Obama (b. 1961). Obama is—wait for it—only six years older than my son Jeff. Being older than the president was hard to accept. Being old enough to be the president's Dad is flat-out scary.

When I was young, facts were jealously guarded treasures. Salespeople controlled their clients by withholding crucial facts. Today, thanks to Google and the myriad other Internet search engines, deep, dark secret facts are dirt cheap commodities.

What's rare today is the ability to put freebie facts into context. Empathy is also mighty scarce. *WTEG* is chock-full of context and empathy. It isn't an "as told to" book. This is an "I understand exactly how you feel because

I've been there and done that" book. There is no hidden agenda. I offer suggestions, not directives; options, not orders.

When you finish *WTEG*, you'll have new ideas about how to play your endgame. What you do with these ideas is up to you. The truth will set you free. Making reality your new best friend will greatly increase your odds of winning the endgame.

PART ONE

AGING WISELY

Chapter 1

STAYING POWER

After reading this chapter, you'll know how to estimate where you are on the continuum between birth and death. Then you can determine your staying power. The more staying power you have, the more risks you can take. And vice versa.

Middle age isn't a one-size-fits-all tube sock. Your middle age won't be the same as mine, because you and I will have different life spans. Your middle age depends on how long you live, not how long I live. It's the middle of your life, not mine.

Latter day Ponce de Leóns want to extend middle age by making 70 the new 50, a beguiling prospect for geezers like me. Try as I might, I can't choke down the Kool-Aid gushing from their ersatz fountain of youth. Extrapolating this specious premise makes 140 the new 100.

Sure. You betcha.

CHEERY FACTOID

The three stages of life are youth, middle age, and "You look great."

When the 2010 U.S. Census was taken, 53,364 Americans were centenarians. There are more members in the Century Club now than ever before. Depending on your gender, you'll either be delighted or despondent to hear that better than four out of five of those centenarians were of the female persuasion.

The Census Bureau helpfully reduced those 53,364 hardy souls down to a more manageable 1.73 centenarians per every 10,000 Americans. Don't reach for your abacus. I converted that into an even more useful stat. Your odds of living to 100 are 5,780 to 1. On the bright side, this proves someone occasionally makes it into the Century Club. It might be you. Bon chance.

I fearlessly forecast that neither of us will live to 140. Death drew a line in the sands of time beyond which *Homo sapiens* seemingly cannot pass. According to Wikipedia, the world record holder for oldest verifiable age is supercentenarian Frenchwoman Jeanne Calment. She survived 122 years plus another 164 days for good measure before dying of natural causes in 1997. Thus far in recorded history one person out of Earth's many billions almost made it to 122 and a half. So much for 140 being the new 100.

Our life span isn't increasing, but our life expectancy is. Americans added three decades to our average life expectancy in the twentieth century. Most of this increase was due to medical advances that slashed U.S. mortality rates for women during childbirth and children in early infancy. The weaker sex's

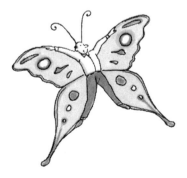

average life expectancy hovers around 81, versus 76 for us big strong guys. This tidbit comes from a report released in October 2014 by the National Center for Health Statistics (NCHS)—part of the U.S. Centers for Disease Control and Prevention (CDC) in Atlanta. Mother Nature built ladies like Sherman tanks to withstand the rigors of childbirth. By comparison to the truly stronger sex, men are fragile butterflies.

Male or female, the longer you live the better are your odds of living even longer. U.S. life expectancy is slowly increasing due to improved medical care, effective vaccination campaigns, and successful public health measures against smoking. If you're still frolicking on the north side of grass at age 65, the CDC estimates guys have about eighteen years of life left and gals approximately twenty more years.

But, don't bet your life on another thirty-year jump in U.S. life expectancy during this century. We've already picked the low-hanging fruit. Until we find cures for cancer, heart disease, stroke, and the other scourges plaguing us, that won't happen. Heart disease and cancer alone account for more than half of all deaths.

And, interestingly, the graying of America has increased the death rate from Alzheimer's disease and suicide. Bette Davis nailed it when she said that old age ain't no place for sissies.

These figures from the Census Bureau and CDC are statistics, not guarantees. If you want to see how charmingly capricious Death is, check the Afterword. You'll find lots of famous folks who moved on while I was writing *WTEG*. I culled these celebrity corpses from obituaries, the factual articles written by newspaper reporters. To get a truly random slice of death, study obits. They're proof positive that having beaucoup bucks and the best care big bucks can buy does not guarantee you'll live to a ripe old age. Some celebs beat the odds. Some didn't. C'est la vie.

Do not try to predict life expectancy by checking the paid death notices in your local newspaper. Unlike obituaries, death notices aren't hard news. They're paid memorial announcements written by bereaved family members, friends, or funeral homes. The In Memory section of your paper doesn't list everyone who dies in your vicinity. It's a cash register that rings every time grief-stricken

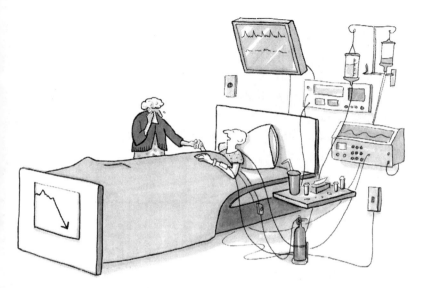

"I'm beginning to think I might be approaching middle age."

folks pay to run a memorial classified ad mourning their loss.

I suspect some people who mistakenly believe 70 is the new 50 have been unduly influenced by paid death notices that disproportionately memorialize ladies and gents in their 80s, 90s, or the Century Club. To get what the esteemed Joe Friday calls a fact, check the CDC's annual life expectancy report, census data, or obituaries. Which neatly seg-ues into staying power—how much time you have to bounce back onto your feet financially or physically after fate kicks you in the butt. To calculate your staying power, start by esti-mating where you are now on the continuum between your birth and death.

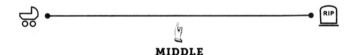

MIDDLE

First, write the year you were born under the baby cradle. Fear not. Your secret is safe—I can't peek.

Now comes the tricky part. Unless you're psychic or currently enjoying free room and board on death row, you don't know when you'll die. Ignore articles that promise you'll live another fifty years if you only eat less than an air fern, exercise more rigorously than Jane Fonda, and visit a plastic surgeon monthly to tweak your rested look.

That's not relentlessly ruthless realism. To age wisely, base your risk management deci-sions on a pragmatic assessment of how much longer you're likely to live. Realism is better than false optimism. Being overly optimistic sets you up to be the next Bambi frozen in the headlights of Fate's semi.

Here's an infallible test to see if you absent-mindedly ambled past the midpoint of your life: double your age. Is anybody twice your age still sipping Champagne? No? Bummers, dear reader. You're definitely more than halfway through your sojourn on lovely planet Earth.

I'll be your canary in the staying power mineshaft. I selected 80 as my bon voyage age. That's six years longer than my Dad lived, but less than the CDC's current life expectancy projection for a guy my age. Plus, 80 is an easy number to work with.

Here's how staying power works. Say I'm 75 now. Times 2 = 150 years. Curses! Using my very own "double your age" test, I'm a dead man walking. One hundred fifty years is longer than even Jeanne Calment lived. I'm waaaaaaaaaaaay past my "sell by" date.

My son Jared, who's thirty years younger than me, graciously volunteered to demonstrate that one man's risk is another's slam dunk when staying power is involved. If I'm 75, Jared is 45.

Times 2 = 90, just past midpoint. In my example, I assume Jared also croaks when he hits 80.

I'm 75/80th (93.75 percent) of the way to checking out. Jared is 45/80th (56.25 percent). That puts me here on the continuum of life. Jared is way back there.

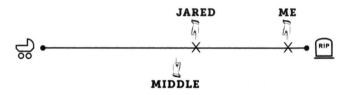

At 75, my staying power (SP) is 80-75 = 5 years. Jared's is 80-45 = 35 years, 7 times longer than mine.

Next year, my SP will be 4 years and Jared's 34—8.5 times longer.

At 77, my SP will be 3 years and Jared's 33—11 times longer.

At 78, my SP will be 2 years and Jared's 32—16 times longer.

At 79, my SP will be 1 year and Jared's 31—31 times longer.

At 80 . . .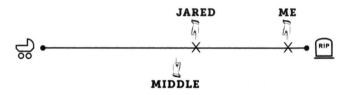

Contrary to what you learned, Einstein's theory is not about the relativity of time. Really, my pal Al was theorizing about the relativity of staying power. Comparing my staying power to Jared's proves Albert's theorem. Staying power zips by me much faster than Jared.

How you play the endgame ultimately depends on your staying power. If you have mucho staying power, you can outlast misfortune. If misfortune has more staying power than you do, don't buy green plantains.

I live in San Francisco. Suppose a quake flattens S.F. tomorrow. It's unlikely my fair city could be restored to pre-quake glory in ten years, but ten years works well in my example, so I'm using it.

Fast forward ten years. If you're ripping pages off a calendar, the decade it took to rebuild San Francisco was identical for Jared and me. Ten years from now, little cable cars once again reach halfway to the stars. Ten years from now, Jared is 55 with twenty-five more years—almost a third of his life—left to savor San Francisco's newly refurbished charms. Jared has staying power.

Not me. My ashes have been blowing in the wind the past five years. The quake turned my golden years into fool's gold. Trying to outlast the rebuilding of San Francisco was insanely risky. I paid dearly because I didn't consider my rapidly declining staying power.

Simone de Beauvoir said that when you age you have a frozen past and an increasingly limited future. As death becomes ever less theoretical, time mutates from friend to enemy. Failure to heed your depleting staying power can have dire consequences.

The gut check question to ask BEFORE disaster strikes is, "Do I have enough staying power to rebuild my life after the coming disaster?" If the answer is "No," you've got a problem. As you'll see in Chapter 5, that problem is manageable.

You have an assignment before reading Chapter 2. Go back to the figures and estimate your staying power. When calculating your staying power, it's OK to increase your bon voyage party age because you're a woman or harken from the deep end of the gene pool. Just be certain the age you select is realistic.

Chapter 2

FINANCING IDEAS FOR HOMEOWNERS

Heed Sardonic Sam Clemens. Mr. C is pointing out the Catch-22 of lending. The best time to get money is when you don't need it. Restating Sam's warning in dire tense, the more desperately you need a loan, the less likely you are to get one.

The #1 pre-retirement financial question for most homeowners is "Should I pay off my mortgage before retiring?" Sounds like a good idea. You'll have less income after you retire, so many financial advisors recommend cutting post-retirement expenses correspondingly. If you own a home, your biggest monthly check is probably your mortgage payment to Friendly Bank. Paying off that loan eliminates your largest expense. It also removes a nagging nightmare—foreclosure if you suffer financial reversals after retiring.

CHEERY FACTOID

A banker is a fellow who lends you his
umbrella when the sun is shining and takes
it back when it begins to rain.

—MARK TWAIN

Hmmm. More cash in your pocket plus
peace of mind. What's not to like? Not so fast,
dear reader. A carpenter would say, "Measure
twice. Cut once." Before hurtling headlong into
a fiscal Waterloo, consider the following hypo-
thetical situation.

Suppose Annie B and I paid off our mortgage before I retired. Further imagine that I
had a massive stroke five years after our gala
mortgage-burning party. After my six-month
stay in Rehabs R Us, Annie B and I visit Friendly
Bank.

"Good morning," I said to the dour lass
who greeted us. "We're here to see Russ."

"Mr. Marinello retired several years ago. I'm Prudence Young-Shark, his replacement."

"Bummers! Russ got us the loan to buy our flats. He refinanced it twice. We love Russ. Ah, well. If he's gone, he's gone.

"I'm bestselling author Ray Brown. The lovely lady pushing my wheelchair is Ann, my ASID (American Society of Interior Designers) interior designer wife. Friendly Bank had our mortgage twenty-five years. We always paid it the first of every month. We were *never* late. We paid off the last $50,000 just before I retired. You still have our checking and savings accounts. You've been our family bank for over thirty years.

"I had a stroke last August. I'll be in this wheelchair the rest of my life. Annie B has many wonderful qualities, but she's too puny to carry me up our front stairs. I need a ramp to get in and out of our flat. We also need to rebuild the shower to accommodate my wheelchair and widen doorways. The contractor estimated it'll cost about $40,000 to do the work.

"We own the flats free and clear. They're in great shape. The real estate agent who came by last week said they're worth around $225,000. That makes the loan-to-value ratio on a $40,000 loan less than 20 percent. Russ would call that a no-brainer.

"Our credit is flawless. How soon will we get the loan, Ms. Young-Shark?"

"I am truly sorry, piteous supplicant. After scanning your income and expense statement, it's as plain as the bulbous nose on your wrinkled face that you don't have enough *disposable* income to repay a $40,000 mortgage. And, just between you and me, Friendly Bank doesn't need any more bad press about kicking old people out of their homes.

"Submitting a loan application would waste your time and—worse yet—my time. Your loan has no chance of being approved. I suggest you develop an appetite for cat food."

Enough frivolity. If you sense I oppose giving Friendly Bank one cent more than you're obligated to pay, you're correct. In a crisis, why put yourself at Friendly Bank's nonexistent sense of mercy to loan you back some of the money you so foolishly prepaid?

Here are two reasons not to pay off your mortgage:

Reason #1—You Break the Liquidity Rule

If you take nothing else away from *WTEG*, remember this—keep your powder dry and your assets liquid. Real property is an illiquid asset. A house isn't a certificate of deposit, share of stock, or bond you can quickly convert into cash. You can't give a real estate agent an order to sell and get equity out of your house in five business days. Even if it's priced to sell, a house usually takes four to six weeks (more in a bad market) to close escrow and cash out.

In my not-so-humble opinion, pouring precious liquid assets into your illiquid house at this stage of your life is wrong, wrong, WRONG. Did I make myself clear?

Unless your Uncle Albert leaves you mega-millions when he kicks the bucket or you win a lottery, where will you get the money to pay off your loan? You'll probably plunder your retirement account or dip into cash you prudently set aside for an emergency.

If you pull big bucks out of your IRA or 401(k) where they're earning tax-deferred income, you'll pay income taxes next year on the withdrawal. The withdrawal may also kick you into a higher tax bracket. If you pour your emergency cash into your house, you're a liquidity crisis waiting to happen. Your fiscal score at this point: Bad options 2. Good options 0.

Discuss the tax consequence of early withdrawal from your retirement account with your financial advisor *before* taking out any money. Instead of paying off your mortgage, you would be wiser to get rid of high interest rate, *non-deductible* consumer debt. Paying off your credit card debt and car loans may save more after-tax money than prepaying your mortgage.

As hard as it is to get cash to pay off your loan, it may be infinitely harder—if not impossible—to pull equity out of your house in an emergency. After you pay off the mortgage, you'll be living in a gold mine without a pickax.

True, you won't have interest payments if you pay off your mortgage. But, with interest rates low now, that won't be a huge windfall. Refinancing, which I cover later in this chapter, is a better option.

Here's the second reason paying off your loan is a bad idea:

Reason #2—You Break the Diversification Rule

Don't put all your fiscal eggs in one basket. If you offer to pay off your loan, Friendly Bank will grab the cash. After you own your house free and clear, you're the only one with skin in the game—a lonely place to be.

The housing market is cyclical. Given today's improved real estate market in much of the U.S., you may think your home's value is rock solid. How quickly you've forgotten the fog of fear that blanketed residential real estate in 2008 when the market dived due south.

By the first quarter of 2011, after nearly three years of short sales and foreclosures, 28 percent of U.S. homeowners were "underwater" (they owed more on their mortgages than their homes were worth). Nearly ten million Americans were still underwater in April 2014—almost six years after the housing bubble burst. Until the market recovered by absorbing distressed properties in your neighborhood, your home's value had the consistency of Jell-O.

Just because *you* always paid your loan on time doesn't mean everyone else did. If a house in your neighborhood went into foreclosure because its owners didn't make *their* loan payments, that foreclosure pulled down your home's value. If you had a home equity line of credit, Friendly Bank could yank it or slash your credit limit to reflect you home's reduced value. I call this bushwhacking by proximity.

The Ghastly Recession spawned a pernicious phenomenon I'd never seen before—strategic defaults. Suppose Gordon Gekko, Oliver Stone's antihero in *Wall Street,* owned the house next door to you. Because his house was deeply underwater, Gekko decided to strategically default (renege on his loan) *even though he could easily afford to make his loan payments.*

I know you'd never renege on a loan. However, the possibility that you *might* is all that matters to Friendly Bank. When Gordy callously opted to cut and run, his strategic default reduced your home's value. More bushwhacking by proximity.

Enough about diversification. Let's discuss uncertainty. Red-hot market or rotten, buyers vehemently abhor overpaying for property. Conversely, sellers vehemently abhor "giving their house away." If neither buyer nor seller gives an inch, no sale.

Uncertainty kills deals. In 2011, no one knew with certainty how deep the home price freefall would be nor when prices would recover.

Buyers *thought* the worst was yet to come and made lowball offers to protect against further price erosion. Sellers *thought* the worst was over and asked more for their houses than the market would bear. It was a classic stalemate.

In a battle between pessimists and optimists, pessimists prevail. It's the golden rule. Whoever has gold rules. Pessimistic buyers and pessimistic banks ruled the 2011 housing market.

Don't kid yourself. Because today's market is strong doesn't mean it will always be strong. Rigid thinking can ruin you. *Always* and *never* are inflexible words. They're like mighty oak trees with deep tap roots. When the fierce winds of change blow, inflexible people with *always* and *never* mindsets are uprooted by the storm. They don't survive.

Survivors are flexible. When you try to predict what the future holds in the real estate market (or stock market), use flexible words like *maybe, perhaps,* and *currently.* Outside of death, taxes, and your dog's unconditional love, nothing is forever.

Sewage happens—usually at the worst possible time. Are you absolutely certain sure you'll *never* need the cash you used to pay off your loan for something slightly more important like paying medical expenses or buying food? Mother Nature isn't benign. You'll develop an insatiable craving for cash after Ma slaps you with a flood, tornado, wildfire, quake, or mudslide. Your odds of getting a loan are zip when your house is a pile of rubble or filled with mud or splinters in the wind or a charred spot.

Today's low interest rates offer borrowers a fantastic opportunity. This may be your once-in-a-lifetime chance to get a fixed-rate mortgage (FRM) at a super-low interest rate. Instead of paying off your mortgage, refinance it. A refi will give you liquidity while saving you tens of thousands of dollars of interest charges over the life of your new, improved, lower interest rate loan. Highlight this paragraph in green, the color of all that money you'll save.

Importantly, don't wait until you're ready to retire to refi. These low FRM interest rates won't last forever. Even if they did, what good are low rates if you can't qualify for a loan? Refinance now when you're at the peak of your earning power with bright prospects for more years of employment. Remember—the best time to get a loan is when you don't need one.

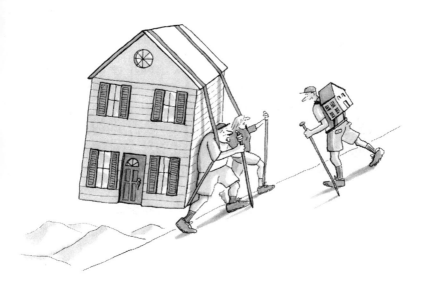

"Retirement's great, isn't it?"

Mortgage rates are currently near historic lows. The 30-year FRM interest rates are around 4.0 percent. Rates on 15-year FRMs are even lower. Your guess is as good as mine as to how long mortgage rates will stay this low. I will, however, state categorically that loan rates can't go much lower. I will state even more categorically that they can go higher. *Much* higher.

Here's some of the context I promised you. In the fall of 1974 (my first year in real estate),

FRM interest rates hit a then-record high of 12 percent before falling back into the 8 percent range. Then, in the early 1980s double-digit inflation reared its ugly head. FRM interest rates went over 18 percent *and stayed over 10 percent for most of the 1980s.* FRM interest rates hovered around 8 to 9 percent throughout the 1990s.

Groucho Marx said he'd never belong to a club that would have him as a member. When loan rates hit 18 percent, buyers everywhere did a Groucho. They wouldn't live in houses they could afford to buy with the tiny mortgages they could qualify for. Pray you never need a loan when loan rates are 18 percent.

There are other gotchas skulking in the shadows. It ain't carved on Mount Rushmore that loan *terms* and *conditions* never change. On the contrary, terms and conditions are *far* more stringent in 2016 than they were ten years earlier. The go-go days when you could get stated-income, no-documentation liar's loans are gone.

Federal regulators cut the maximum amount they insure on Fannie Mae and Freddie Mac loans. That pushed up interest rates on "jumbo" mortgages, those over $417,000. Federal regulators now insist that borrowers make larger down payments, figuring more skin in the game reduces the odds of future foreclosures. Borrowers need higher credit scores and lower debt-to-disposable-income ratios to qualify for loans today.

Whether mortgage rates are near an all-time low or not, refinancing before you retire to increase your liquidity is generally a good idea. Consider that savings account interest rates fluctuate in synch with mortgage rates. Lenders usually maintain roughly a 3 percent spread between mortgage rates and interest paid on savings accounts. With FRM rates near 4 percent now, savings accounts pay about 1 percent. When FRM rates return to the normal 8–9 percent range, savings accounts will pay 5–6 percent. Cash you sock away now will eventually earn a decent return again.

Now let's look at reverse annuity mortgages. RAMs are FHA insured loan products specifically designed for house-rich, cash-poor seniors. If you're at least 62, a RAM lets you borrow against the equity in your home *without making monthly payments.* You can pull equity out in one of three ways:

1. A lump sum payment.
2. Monthly payments based upon your life expectancy.
3. A line of credit you can dip into as needed.

However, you don't get something for nothing. Every month the accrued interest on your RAM is added to the principal amount you originally borrowed. Your loan gets big and bigger because you're paying interest on the principal as well as interest on your accrued interest—exactly the reverse of what happens with a regular mortgage. Hence the name.

You don't repay principal or interest until you either 1) sell the house or 2) move out for more than twelve months or 3) die. If you outlive the actuarial tables or if property values tank, your outstanding loan balance may exceed your house's value when you croak or move out. In that case, the FHA's insurance fund makes up the difference. You or your heirs are off the hook.

If you die or sell under normal circumstances, either you or your estate must repay the principal amount borrowed plus accrued interest. The remaining equity, if any, goes to you or your heirs.

I find it interesting that Wells Fargo, the nation's largest home lender, stopped originating RAMs in June 2011. Wells Fargo said the continued unpredictability of home values made RAMs too risky. Bank of America, the second-largest U.S. home lender, came to the same conclusion earlier that year. If humongous lending institutions like Wells Fargo and Bank of America thought RAMs are too risky, what are the implications for ordinary mortals like thee and me?

I am not a RAM fan because

RAMs are complicated. The RAM must be the first mortgage on your house. If you have an existing loan, you must pay it off before you get a RAM. No matter how much your house is worth, the amount you can borrow is based upon a predetermined percentage of its value not to exceed a

$625,000 cap. The percentage you can borrow also depends upon your age and then-current interest rates. There are many other terms and conditions. Due to their complexity, you can't get a RAM until you meet with a FHA approved loan counselor. You pay a fee for this mandatory consultation whether you ultimately get the RAM or not.

RAMs are expensive. The FHA charges a one-time up-front mortgage insurance premium based on your house's appraised value. You also pay *annual* mortgage insurance premiums as long as you have the RAM. And you pay the FHA-approved lender who makes the loan an origination fee and closing costs. And, of course, you must keep paying your property taxes, homeowner's insurance, homeowner's association fees, and other normal ownership expenses. Should sewage happen and circumstances force you to move out or you die shortly after incurring these expenses, tough noogie.

RAM interest rates are generally 1 to 1.5 percent higher than what you'd pay if you simply refinanced your mortgage. Compared to refinancing, a RAM is more complicated, more expensive to originate, and has a higher interest rate. What's to like?

RAMs enable you to remain in a house that may no longer be age-appropriate.

RAM or not, you'll have other expenses after you retire. You'll still have to pay for gas and electricity, paint jobs, roof repairs, and other maintenance expenses plus insurance and property tax. Inflation is dormant, not dead. It'll rear its ugly head again, we just don't know when. Trust me—owning a home won't get cheaper after you retire.

Farmers save seed corn from their harvest to plant next year's crop. Trying to decide whether or not to eat seed corn to survive a brutal winter is a dreadful dilemma. Is it better to starve right away or eventually? (The best response to this kind of bleak choice is Jack Benny's reply to the robber who demanded his money or his life: "I'm thinking. I'm thinking.")

Money squirreled away for retirement is financial seed corn. *Cannibalize* aptly describes what you'll do if you spend precious seed corn in a misguided attempt to keep a house you can't afford. If you ignore economic reality, your beloved house will eat every kernel. It has an insatiable appetite for seed corn.

One way to conserve seed corn is to sell your house and rent. If you're fixated on owning rather than renting, at least move to a less-expensive area where you'll get a bigger bang for your housing buck. If you spend too much of your discretionary retirement income keeping a roof over your head, you don't own the house. It owns you. Sooner or later, it will devour you.

Chapter 3

SELLING YOUR HOME

Selling your house might be gut wrenching. Overstaying your welcome can be financially —even literally—deadly. Welcome to devilish dilemma du jour. You have the following alternatives to consider:

Do nothing. My pal Isaac Newton calls this the inertia option. Stay in the house you bought eons ago when your long-departed children were adorable rug rats. Cast a blind eye to the ravages time has wrought on your dream house and you. Dynamic inaction was popular with dodos and dinosaurs.

Rightsize. You want to live in the moment, not the memory. Selling your old dream house frees you to move into an

CHEERY FACTOID

You may love your house,
but it doesn't love you.

age-appropriate home, condo, or retirement community. This isn't downsizing, which has negative connotations of defeat. You're rightsizing into a cornucopia of new, improved life-style options.

Rent. This option eliminates headaches and maximizes financial freedom. After living in your house for years, you want to live on income generated by your equity. Time to let somebody else worry about mowing the grass, raking leaves, shoveling snow, repairing the roof, and all that other tiresome maintenance stuff.

In the next chapter, we look at brick and mortar, post-retirement housing options. In this chapter, we focus on one topic—to sell or not to sell your house. Here's how Annie B and I muddled through it.

We closed escrow on our dream home on April Fool's Day 1978. The two flats we bought were in "original condition." That's Realtor speak for unmitigated disaster. We camped in the lower flat while the upper unit was gutted and rebuilt.

Sixteen hellish months later, we moved into the refurbished 3-bedroom, 2-bath upper unit. No more turf wars. Our sons, Jeff and Jared, each had his own bedroom. The master bedroom overlooking Mountain Lake Park was blissfully quiet. Annie B had transformed great potential into heavenly reality.

Life was idyllic.

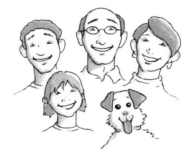

Idyllic is unsustainable.

Bandit, the wonder dog, died on June 29, 1985. We sadly scattered his trustworthy, loyal, and steadfast ashes in the park he loved.

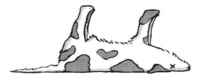

Two months later, Jeff left for his freshman year at college. Heavy sighs from Annie B and me whenever we passed the Jeffrey J Brown Shrine Room, frozen in pristine disarray. To Jared's consternation, we laser-focused our formidable parental energy entirely on him. Jared fled to college in August 1987. Another shrine room. More sighs.

Except for semester breaks and summers when Jeff and Jared graced us with pit stops to eat, sleep, and do laundry, silence enveloped us. Jeff moved out for good in June 1990. Jared departed two years later. For the first time in twenty-five years, Annie B and I were empty nesters.

Walking the same old streets to the same old restaurants to eat the same old food and shop in the same old stores got old fast. We sporadically discussed selling the flats. On a purely intellectual level, we knew two shriveled peas didn't need such a humongous pod.

After vacillating merely six years, we moved into the smaller lower flat. By doing so, we cut the gas and electric bill. We eliminated two flights of stairs. We didn't have to leave our wonderful neighbors or beloved park. We avoided the hassle and expense of selling our house and buying a new one. It was the perfect solution. Like changing deck chairs on the *Titanic*.

Annie B and I were still empty nesters in a family neighborhood. We still trudged the same streets to the same restaurants and shopped in the same stores. Our net worth was still tied up in an illiquid asset. It was a fiscal disaster waiting to happen.

The real reason we didn't sell was inertia. Annie B and I lacked the energy to tackle twenty years of junk jammed into our attic.

Valuable stuff like the rocking chair we lulled the boys to sleep in when they were babies, phonograph records that might be collectors' items someday, and clothes we'd wear again when we lost a few pounds. Junk is bad. Memories are worse.

We couldn't cull life's flotsam and jetsam— report cards, finger painting masterpieces, birthday cards, baby clothes, photographs, Super 8 movies, locks of Jeff and Jared's hair from their first haircuts, baby teeth the Tooth Fairy lovingly collected. Deciding which treasures to keep and which to toss was impossible. It was easier to keep kicking the mess down the road.

Delay is the deadliest form of denial. Ike Newton understood inertia. He said a pile of junk remains at rest unless acted upon by an outside force. Annie B and I wanted to let sleeping junk lie. I didn't know then that junk only hibernates so long.

The metamorphosis from happy homeowner into "motivated" seller occurs when your dream home becomes nightmarishly inhospitable. You have a stroke, your wife breaks a hip, or the mighty Mississippi floods you out. Whatever.

When the trap springs, you don't have the luxury of time to wait for the best offer. You take what you can get, dump your junk, and move. So long, neighborhood. Hello, victimhood. You do *not* want this to happen to you.

I'm blush to confess that moving into the lower flat delayed our departure another eight years. Like *The Shadow,* inertia has the power to cloud your mind. It lulls you into false complacency. We'd still be there if Annie hadn't heard about an apartment for rent that had an unobstructed view sweeping from the Golden Gate Bridge to the Bay Bridge. For Annie B and me, it was love at first sight again. Love, not misfortune, broke inertia's deadly paralysis.

We called a real estate agent while driving home. Monday was Memorial Day. Our For Sale sign went up Tuesday. The flats sold quickly, and we moved on to our next adventure. By now you're probably saying, "Is there a point here somewhere, Ray?" Yup, two:

1. Your shelter requirements change as your family evolves.
2. Selling your dream home is easier in theory than in fact.

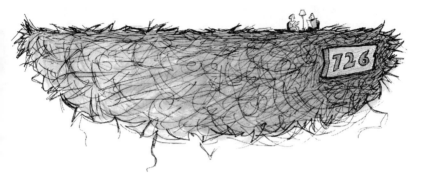

As a snake sheds its outgrown skin, you must shed your house when it outlives its usefulness. I know it isn't easy. Annie B and I lingered on fourteen years *after* our fledglings flew the nest.

I'll tell you a secret. Good real estate agents understand the difference between a *condition* and an *objection*. A condition can't be defeated with additional information. An objection, on the other hand, can be overcome with more info. When you say "No" to good agents, they assume you're objecting because you don't have enough information *yet* to say "Yes."

If, for instance, your spouse is permanently bedridden, nothing an agent says will tempt you to buy a house with a stunning view from the master bedroom on the third floor. When you tell your agent not to show you houses with stairs, that's a condition—not an objection.

Here are objections I hear from empty nesters when I recommend they sell their obsolete dream house and rightsize into an age-appropriate replacement home:

We love our neighbors. There's no law against visiting your neighbors whenever you want after you move. You aren't losing your old neighbors, you're gaining new ones you may grow to love every bit as much—perhaps even more.

We love the neighborhood. The 'hood ain't going anywhere. Like neighbors, you can visit your old haunts whenever you wish.

We're OK where we are—finding a new butcher, baker, and candlestick maker is more hassle than it's worth. You're in a rut.

Do you still read *The Saturday Evening Post* and watch silent movies? Get a life.

Our house isn't perfect, but we know what we've got. Translation, "Better a devil we know than an angel we don't." You'd rather put up with your house's flaws than move. You'll be fine as long as you keep patching the leaky roof, keep propping up the fence so it doesn't blow over, and keep bundling up when icy winds blast through the front windows. Oh, yeah. And as long as you can still make it up all those stairs.

Where will we put our stuff if we move to a smaller place? Donating clothes you'll never wear again to Goodwill, shredding twenty years of tax returns you're keeping "just in case," and dumping junk in your attic is incredibly liberating. If you don't winnow your treasures now, your kids will when you're gone. As in dead.

We'll pay capital gains tax. Probably not. The U.S. median sale price for an existing single-family home was nearly $230,000 in the fourth quarter of 2015, according to the National Association of Realtors. (Half the houses in America sold for more than the median price, half sold for less.) As Eric Tyson and I note in *House Selling for Dummies,* single taxpayers can realize up to $250,000 of profit on the sale of their house without paying any federal income tax thanks to the Taxpayer Relief Act passed by Congress in 1997. That increases to $500,000 of profit for married couples.

Given this generous exemption, most folks won't pay much, if any, capital gains tax as long as the house was their primary residence for at least two of the five years immediately preceding the sale. Congress delights in tax code tinkering. Discuss the after-tax consequences of selling with your tax advisor before putting your house on the market.

We intend to will the house to our children. BIG mistake! A better way to handle this explosive scenario is to sell the house after you die and distribute the proceeds of sale to your kids. In one fell swoop, you'll eliminate real or imagined complaints about favoritism as well as the possibility of a pernicious multigenerational family feud.

Punch inertia in the nose. Be fiscally ruthless. Rightsize when your house no longer satisfies your needs. Or sell it, invest the proceeds of sale, and rent. Use income from your investments to help pay the rent. Either option beats letting inertia ruin your life.

With a nod to Ecclesiastes, for everything including the endgame there is a season:

A time to buy your dream home and a time to rightsize.

A time to take risks and a time to be prudent.

A time to own and a time to rent.

A time to live independently and a time for assisted living.

If you don't control your destiny, it will control you. Doing nothing isn't an option. Passivity spawns victims. The clock is ticking. Time will either be your friend or your enemy. Victor or victim? Your choice.

Chapter 4

ENDGAME HOUSING ALTERNATIVES

Deciding where to live after you retire is difficult. If you're in a long-term relationship, it's emotional nitro because you must also consider your partner's wishes. Some folks make the decision even tougher by asking, "Where will I live *for the rest of my life?"*

Good news. You have an inalienable right to move as often as you wish. Given the expense and aggravation of moving, only masochists willingly move if they don't have to. For the rest of us, it's comforting to remember we can move again—and even again—if move we must.

Let's start by examining hot buttons. Thanks to my previous incarnation as a real estate broker, I know that people don't buy *houses.* They buy *hot buttons*—features that appeal to them—and the rest of the house tags along for the ride.

CHEERY FACTOID

If taken while driving,
naps prevent old age.

Your present house's hot button may've been a chef's kitchen or a sunken living room with a natural stone fireplace or an enormous backyard. Then again, it could've been an external factor such as an easy commute to work or proximity to a stellar grade school. Endgame buyers have different hot buttons than first-time buyers:

Instead of buying to be near a school, now you want to be near your grandchildren.

Rather than building equity, you want to cash out and live on your equity.

Given your newfound concern about vulnerability and diminishing staying power, you've decided it's time to relocate out of harm's way.

Feel free to add your favorite hot buttons to my list. Keep in mind that pushing hot buttons will trigger a seismic shift in your life-style.

Beware, too, of mobile hot buttons. If cozying up to those adorable grandchildren is your hot button, remember that rug rats tag along when their parents move. Think twice before becoming a camp follower. Rather than relocating every time your grandkids do, buy a plane ticket when you need to replenish your stock of unconditional love.

I thoughtfully cut the multitude of end-game housing options down to four:

Option # 1—Stay Put

If you're an empty nester rattling around in your dream home, staying put is your worst option for the reasons noted in Chapter 3. If you haven't read it yet, whose fault is that?

When I was a kid growing up in Yakima, I ran innovative ideas by Mom. Sometimes she blessed my plan; more often than not, Mom lovingly listed the many flaws in my scheme. If I refused to heed her sage advice, she locked her big brown eyes on mine and ominously said, "Fine!" Mom waited till I blinked, then droned part two of her dreaded curse, "It's on *your* head, Raymond." Fair warning, dear reader. If you opt to stay put, it's on *your* head.

Option #2—Rightsize into Another Ownership Property

Ownership opportunities are available in almost as many varieties as Baskin-Robbins ice cream. You can rightsize into any of these delicious options.

Detached Single-Family Dwelling (SFD)

Though your new castle is probably a tad tinier, you're still lord and master of all you survey. As proud owner, you're in complete control. No need to worry about a landlord jacking up your rent or kicking you out. Nor do you need permission to paint the living room in your school colors or bring home a pup or two.

You're da boss. Wait. There's more. Dumping that empty nest for a sleeker, less expensive home lets you

Free up the lazy equity frozen in your ancestral manor. If you spend less on your new casa than you get selling your old one, you'll have cash to invest. The income can then offset some of your living expenses. Remember not to put all your new financial eggs in one basket.

Slash operating expenses. My buddy Ben Franklin says a penny saved is a penny earned. Pennies, schmennies. We're talking big bucks. A smaller, more energy efficient home will be cheaper to heat and cool. You'll pay less for insurance and property taxes, too.

Enjoy a safer, healthier life-style. When you rightsize, go all the way. Move to a benign haven where homes are less expensive, the cost of living is lower, winters are milder, summers are cooler, and never is heard discouraging words like *tornado,* *earthquake,* or *hurricane.* Get out of harm's way while the getting is good.

Anticipate the inevitable. Falls happen. Rightsize into a home without stairs. Nix places with an attic or basement you might not be able to use someday. If your new home isn't wheelchair accessible, someday it may become functionally obsolete (Realtor speak for uninhabitable). Tough love, dear reader.

Don't overdo rightsizing.

A couple in our apartment building began slipping into infirmity soon after we moved in. Dementia wasn't the culprit; 'twas the relentless ravages of aging. In time they needed help getting on and off the john, bathing, and cooking. Climbing into and out of bed became a death defying feat.

They had long-term care insurance (do you?), but no room in their apartment for a live-in caregiver. Eventually, those nice folks had to move. Not easy to do in your 80s. Be sure your new digs can accommodate a live-in caregiver if need be. Enough said.

Condominium or Cooperative Apartments

The Disadvantages.

Rightsizing from a house into a condo or co-op requires the ability to play well with others. If you're too blithe a spirit to cope with the rules, regulations, and life-style changes communal living imposes on you, skip this section. You will not fit in. (Note I didn't say "probably won't"—there isn't a scintilla of wiggle room.) If I haven't scared you off, read on.

Condos and co-ops are less private than detached SFDs. There will probably be some noise pollution. After all, you share walls, floors, and ceilings with other owners. Did I mention you can't amble around buck ass naked in common areas? If your bod is as bad as mine, that's not a deal killer. After a certain age, clothes are good.

Condos and co-ops are legally and fiscally complex. You *aren't* lord and master of all you survey. You co-own it with others. Read legal documents, bylaws, and the budget line by line before buying. Consult an attorney if you have questions about what various documents mean or how they affect you. Scrutinize the last three years' operating budgets and financial statements. Run if you find frequent homeowner's association (HOA) dues hikes or special assessments. Are many owners delinquent paying HOA dues? Harking back to Chapter 2, ask if there have been short sales, strategic defaults, or foreclosures.

Condos and co-ops are restrictive. Like fences, good legal docs make good neighbors. When lots of people live in close proximity, you need rules to maintain civility and order. Conditions, Covenants, and Restrictions (CC&Rs) specify constraints such as the type of window and floor coverings you must have in your unit; whether you can have a pet; alterations you can/can't make; how often you may entertain and how many of your pals can attend your party. I could go on, but you get the idea. Too many rules turn a happy home into a prison. It's almost impossible to change CC&Rs. Don't buy into an overly restrictive complex.

The Advantages.

If you can handle communal living, rightsizing into a condo or co-op offers the ownership advantages enumerated in the SFD section plus these bonus goodies:

Bigger bang for your buck. Compare the purchase price of a two-bedroom condo or co-op to a two-bedroom SFD in the same neighborhood. The cost per livable square foot will likely be 20 to 30 percent lower for the condo or co-op. Sharing building expenses with other owners beats buying it all by yourself.

Lower operating expenses. Say you own a condo in a fifty-unit building. If the building needs a new roof, the cost is prorated with the other forty-nine owners. Matter of fact, you split all common area costs with the other owners, such as an exterior paint job, cleaning the entryway carpet, or replacing broken windows. There's economic strength in numbers.

No maintenance headaches. When you live in a condo or co-op, you won't fret about having a heart attack mowing the lawn when it's 110 degrees in the shade or shoveling snow during a blizzard. Nor will you fracture your skull falling off the roof while clearing the rain gutters. The apartment gods invented homeowner's associations to handle maintenance aggravations.

More amenities. How many of your pals own a SFD with a twenty-four-hour doorman, tennis courts, a swimming pool, and exercise facilities? Darn few, I wager. When owners in a condo or co-op complex share the costs, impossible dreams become reality. Imagine the hedonistic delight of telling the doorman to collect your mail and sign for packages while you're visiting your grandchildren or touring the Taj Mahal.

Option #3—Rightsize into a Rental

Why did Annie B and I decide to rent? We live in San Francisco, which is overdue for a big quake. We accept this risk with the same equanimity that other folks accept the possibility of occasional floods, tornadoes, hurricanes, or blizzards. Paradise flawed. Annie B and I weren't overly concerned about being injured or killed in a quake. We were, however, deeply disturbed that most of our life savings was tied up in the equity we have in our flats. We knew property values will likely tank after a big quake. It became more and more difficult for us to reconcile the joy of living in San Francisco with the threat of impending impoverishment.

Our plight is yours when you live in a disaster prone area. If most of your net worth is the equity in your house, the next cataclysmic natural disaster could wipe you out. Will you live long enough for property values to recover? How do you feel about spending your golden years dining on construction dust during a protracted reconstruction?

To stay in a disaster prone area with financial impunity, Annie B and I sold our flats and became renters. Here's why:

Selling the flats freed 100 percent of our equity to invest out of harm's way. If a big one creams San Francisco tomorrow, the lovely ladies who own our building have a problem. Not us. We can stick around after the quake or fly the coop without economic consequences.

Renting in a large apartment building gave us the same amenities we'd have in a large condo or co-op complex. We live in a wheelchair accessible, elevator build-ing with a twenty-four-hour doorman. We don't have any maintenance headaches.

Renting gave us a bigger bang for our housing buck. This sounds ridiculous, but it's true in Washington, D,C., Manhattan, Ft. Lauderdale, Honolulu, or any other place with expensive real estate. Comparing our rent to what we'd have to pay in homeown-er's association dues, principal, interest, and property taxes to buy a comparable SFD, condo, or co-op, we're ahead renting.

True, we don't get the appreciation in our apartment's value. The tradeoff is we didn't have to make a big down payment. That cash is earning money for us elsewhere. And while we don't get a tax deduction for our rent, we don't need as much tax shelter now because we have less income to shelter. If Bill Devlin, our peerless CPA, isn't upset, we're OK.

Option #4—Rightsize into Happy Acres

Seniors used to be warehoused in dreary old folks' homes until they kicked the bucket. Not anymore. Now Happy Acres has a moniker that befits its new elegance—a Continuing Care Retirement Community (CCRC). I was first exposed to a CCRC in 1988 when my pal Ray Jones moved into The Peninsula Regent.

Even more important than its elegant furnishing and fine dining was The Peninsula Regent's promise to Ray—that when his health failed they'd provide a seamless, tiered continuum of care to surmount the inevitable ravages of aging. Color me skeptical. Talk's cheap.

Ray J put The Peninsula Regent to the test when he was diagnosed with pancreatic cancer in 1990. From diagnosis to death nine months later, their stellar staff gave Ray the tenderest of loving care. He wanted for nothing and suffered not. Thanks to them, Ray J slipped ever so gently into that good night. He died as well as anyone I've ever seen. (Don't take my word about CCRCs. You can see what one looks like for yourself. The Peninsula Regent is conveniently located at peninsularegent.com. If a picture is worth one thousand words, their website is an encyclopedia. Use it as a template when looking for CCRCs in your area.)

Rejoice that you're coming of age now. You can join a CCRC while you're still vigorous, healthy, and capable of living independently. You'll maintain your active life-style and pursue whatever interests tickle your fancy. Life is good. Somewhat further down the yellow brick road, life may become less good. If, like Ray J, your health fails, you're covered. You'll move into assisted living. Some CCRCs even offer skilled nursing and medical care on-site.

Birth to earth care isn't cheap, mind you. Some—not all—CCRCs charge you a hefty entry fee. You'll also have monthly charges for meals, housekeeping service, transportation service, educational and social programs, wellness and fitness courses, etc., etc., and etc. The more services you use, the more you pay. That's fair. How much you ultimately pay depends upon a variety of factors. Here are a few:

1. The current state of your health.

2. Where you live (the higher the cost of living in your locale, the more expensive the CCRC).

3. Whether you rent or buy.

4. The type of housing (SFD, condo, apartment) you select.

5. How many residents (just you, or you and your spouse/partner) live in the CCRC.

6. Whether you get a deluxe extended contract that covers unlimited assisted living, medical treatment, and skilled nursing or an a la carte, fee-for-service contract.

AARP is a treasure trove of information about CCRCs. Among other things, AARP urges you to be sure the CCRC you select will remain in operation and stay financially stable as long as you live. They suggest spending a few days in the CCRC before signing up to be sure it's right for you. Last, but not least, they recommend that your attorney review the CCRC contract before you pledge your troth to it.

AARP is the best resource I've found for info about every aspect of aging. Knowing how lazy I am, you won't be surprised to learn that I have no intention of reinventing any of their perfectly good wheels. Check out AARP at www.aarp.org. You *will* learn a thing or two.

Now for a gut check on the concept of moving into Happy Acres. Even if price is no object, I know many otherwise delightful, intelligent folks who are viscerally opposed to ever, *ever* residing in a CCRC, no matter how deluxe. This isn't idle speculation. I live with one. "Just shoot me," Annie B hissed as we left a dementia facility after visiting our dear friend Bob, a once-gifted guy now being sliced and diced by

Alzheimer's. Seeing the eviscerated shell that once was Bob always depressed us.

My wife is irrevocably unwilling to abide in Happy Acres. She doesn't want to be surrounded by peers in varying stages of decomposition. She doesn't want to watch their health deteriorate. She doesn't want to see them regress from walking to walkers to wheelchairs to bedridden. She doesn't want to watch buckets kicked one by one.

Ask not for whom the bells toll. The Ferragamo will be on the other foot in the highly unlikely event that Annie B changes her mind. *The Happy Acres Paradox* is the 21st century's version of *Catch-22*. Here's the screenplay:

Act 1. Happy Acres pursues Annie B and me with the unbridled enthusiasm of a golden retriever pup. We brusquely reject their blandishments. We're far too young to cast our lot with a coven of coots.

Act 2. Excrement happens. A stroke strikes. Ministering to me 24/7 soon wears Annie B down to a nubbin of her formerly vibrant

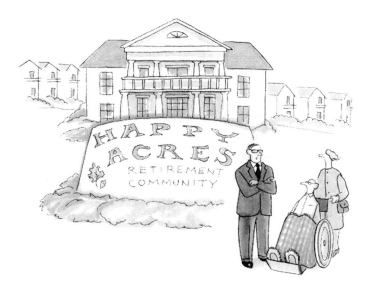

*"I'm sorry, we only welcome healthy, vibrant residents.
I suggest you try Crappy Acres."*

self. Hats in hand, we humbly beseech Happy Acres for admittance.

Act 3. Happy Acres raises the drawbridge, fills its moat with alligators and threatens to pour boiling oil on us if we miraculously make it across. Too late the fog of ignorance dissipates. At last we understand how the game is played. As long as you don't need to get into Happy Acres, you can. If you need to get in, you can't.

That wasn't *my* stroke. It was *our* stroke. What adversely affects one of us, adversely affects both of us. Sweet Annie B and I are, for better or for worse, in sickness and in deteriorating health, inextricably joined at the hip till death do us part.

Don't confuse Happy Acres with the Statue of Liberty. Happy Acres does *not* welcome the tired, the poor, the huddled masses. Happy Acres is a for-profit business. The best time—in fact, only time—to get into Happy Acres is *before* you need to. Wrap your mind around this thought before dismissing Happy Acres as a place decrepit people go to die. The folks in a CCRC toddle off to their big sleep with more grace, companionship, and dignity than loners who shuffle to a solitary end making noise no one hears.

Happy Acres isn't a place you go to die. It's where you go to live better longer. IF Annie B dies before I do, I'll move into Happy Acres. IF Happy Acres will have me.

Two big IFs.

Chapter 5

RISK MANAGEMENT

***Vulnerability* is increased susceptibility** to injury or harm. You'll spot signs of increased vulnerability after you turn 60. People mumble more, menus are harder to read, the ground is farther away and harder when you fall, your muscles get flabby, and your steel-trap mind turns into a colander. There are other red flags, but they slipped through my colander.

Boomers born in 1964 turned 50 in 2014. That means most of the youngest class of boomers now have more of their lives behind them than ahead of them. The oldest class of boomers (born 1946) is already getting Medicare benefits. Connect the dots. Vulnerability is roaring toward you.

Running out of time is as bad as physical decline. As noted in Chapter 1, the older you get, the less time you have before dying to get back on your feet literally or financially after

CHEERY FACTOID

The odds for poop plopping double if you're in a relationship. It doesn't matter which one of you is nailed by a rabid rabbit or heart attack, you're both adversely affected. Vulnerability doesn't play favorites.

misfortune smacks you around. Hopeless? Not if you manage the Fearsome Four Risks.

Risk #1—Genetic Risk

If you're blessed with incredible genes like Winston Churchill, you're almost invulnerable. As U.K. Prime Minister from 1940 to 1945, Winnie had a rather stressful job. He was an insomniac; was overly fond of whisky and sodas; smoked like a peat fire; and was more than a tad tubby. Truth is, he'd eat anything that didn't eat him first. Winston was the poster boy for an unhealthy life-style, yet he survived to 90.

If you emerged from the shallow end of the gene pool, you entered the world genetically predisposed to an early demise from cancer, Parkinson's disease, stroke, heart disease, obesity, ALS, diabetes, liver disease, early onset Alzheimer's, kidney failure, or some other malicious malady. DNA happens. Your unique combination of genetic risks was etched into your DNA that marvelous moment you were conceived. If you had the foresight to pick the right Mom and Dad, you're golden. If not, descending into deep depression at this late date won't help. This might:

As he's done every Friday since his bar mitzvah, Abe went to Temple. His prayer began, "Hello, God. It's me, Abe. You know I always faithfully followed your Commandments. Now I'm 85. Even my aches have aches. I won't live much longer.

"I've been poor all my life. That never bothered me. I figured if poor was your will, fine by me. I've never asked you for anything for myself. But it would be nice to leave my children and grandchildren a little something from Papa. So, God, please let me win the lottery. Thank you. Amen."

Next Friday, "Hello, God. It's me, Abe. It's been a week. I haven't won the lottery yet. Please don't forget your obedient servant. Thank you. Amen."

After six months of unanswered prayers, Abe cried out in despair, "Lord. Why hast thou forsaken me?"

Golden light and heavenly music filled the Temple. A deep, benevolent voice implored, "Meet me halfway, Abe. Buy a ticket."

Too subtle? You ain't going to get a free wallow in fatalism because you don't have Winnie's DNA. Don't waste precious time cursing the lousy genes fate bestowed upon you.

You gotta put skin in the game to win. Here are things *you* can do to increase your odds of winning the endgame:

Get periodic physical exams.
Don't surrender to predestination. Be proactive. Monitor the pesky genetic devils incubat-

ing within. As you get older, add a doctor with geriatric skills to your medical team.

Cancer, heart disease, strokes, and many other maladies are age-related. More and more bodily functions go out of warranty as we get older. If you're a guy, for instance, your odds of having prostate cancer when you're 80 are about 50-50 according to John Fletcher, my primary care doc. He said most guys over 80 die *with* prostate cancer, but not *from* it. John assured me something else will probably kill me first.

Comforting.

A physical isn't a game of *I've Got a Secret*. It's not in my best interests to keep *any* secrets from John. He dismisses most things with, "Don't worry about that, Ray. It's a big nothing." Every now and then, however, John says, "That's something we should check out." And we do. Solving a problem starts with discovering you have one.

According to Alzheimer's Association, one out of eight Americans has Alzheimer's by age 65. Guy or gal, your likelihood of developing it after 65 doubles every five years. Should you survive to 85, your odds of having Alzheimer's are 50-50. There is a bright side. If you develop Alzheimer's, you can watch *It's A Wonderful Life* again for the first time.

You also need eye exams.

According to Dr. Michael Turan, my ophthalmologist, cataracts, glaucoma, and macular degeneration sneak up on you when you're not looking (sorry). Get annual eye exams.

Get a colonoscopy.

Physicals and eye exams aren't enough. Our friends at the CDC recommend having a colonoscopy every ten years. According to a study released by the American Cancer Society in 2012, colorectal cancer is the second leading cause of cancer-related death in America. If everyone 50 or older was screened regularly, at least 60 percent of these deaths could be avoided. The five-year survival rate is about 90 percent if you spot colorectal cancer early.

The CDC recommends men and women begin having colonoscopies at age 50 and get follow-up exams every ten years until you're in your 70s. If colorectal cancer runs in your family, ask your doctor about being tested more frequently. The CDC says one out of three U.S. adults is NOT getting screened for colorectal cancer. If you're that person, dear reader, please ponder this. Which is worse—a slow, agonizing death from colorectal cancer or a day devoted to cleansing your colon (you know what I mean) followed by a colonoscopy?

These exams let doctors monitor your vital signs while you're healthy. After establishing your baselines, it's easier to spot things that go amiss. Your doc can treat what ails you while the problem is relatively minor. Because you're proactive, time is your friend—not your enemy. If you're flexible enough, pat yourself on the back.

Good health is more precious than gold. Don't squander it.

Risk #2—Natural Disaster

Japan's earthquake and tsunami that occurred on March 11, 2011, was a gruesome demonstration of Mother Nature's power. The quake was horrific. It paled compared to the ensuing tsunami's near total devastation. Two years after this epic one-two punch, the body count was

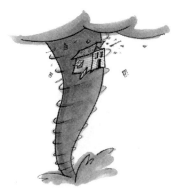

up to nineteen thousand dead or missing. Another three hundred thousand displaced survivors were still living in *temporary* housing.

You can run, but you can't hide. Depending on your zip code, there's a flood, tornado, hurricane, quake, wildfire, cyclone, drought, tsunami, avalanche, blizzard, landslide, volcanic eruption, hailstorm, or mudslide lurking in your future. However, this may make you feel slightly better: Statistically speaking, natural disasters are usually more disruptive than deadly.

The number of folks killed or injured in a tsunami or quake, for example, is relatively small compared to the multitudes who suddenly find themselves homeless. This is, of course, hollow comfort if you're the hapless soul swept out to sea or crushed when your house fell on you. Statistics don't bleed.

Be proactive about natural disasters.

With a tip of my ten-gallon hat to Ross Perot, worrying about your next natural disaster is no more useful than trying to teach a pig how to whistle. It annoys the pig and wastes your time. If you can't sleep because you're fretting about the next disaster, either of these options is better than sleeping pills: 1) Get out of harm's way or 2) Cut your financial risk and increase your post-disaster options by converting yourself from homeowner to renter.

If you're determined to live in a disaster prone area because you love it, fine by me. At least promise me that you'll remain vigilant. *What* you say about the probability of the next disaster can lull you into a false sense of security.

Here's my pop quiz to see if you're in disaster denial mode: When I ask, "Are you ready for your next natural disaster?" do you reply, "*IF* we have a flood, hurricane, tornado, whatever?" or "*WHEN* we have a . . . ?" Grade your own test. No curve here—it's either A or F.

Ask yourself, "What can I do now to minimize my physical and financial exposure and maximize my favorable options when the next disaster strikes?" Don't kid yourself. If you live in harm's way, natural disaster may only be a few heartbeats away.

Put together an emergency kit and prepare an evacuation plan.

Organized disaster relief may not arrive for several days after Mother Nature messes with you. Don't depend on the kindness of strangers. Realistically, you are your own first responder.

Be prepared to take care of yourself for a few days after catastrophe strikes. Have a home emergency kit stocked with three gallons of water and a three-day supply of food *per family member* plus a first-aid kit, crank-operated flashlight, and radio with spare batteries. Check with your local Red Cross chapter for other items you should put in your disaster kit. Learn basic first aid techniques and CPR.

When disaster strikes, you might not have a home to come back to. Keep emergency kits in your car and at work. Select a safe haven where your family can gather after the disaster. Identify a local contact and an out-of-area contact your family can call to find out where you are and how you're doing.

Staying power isn't carved in stone.
Recalculate yours annually to be sure your long-term survival plan is still viable. Be brutally honest. Your tipping point arrives when you're not sure you'll live long enough to survive rebuilding after a disaster.

Which is worse—moving preemptively in anticipation of a disaster that doesn't occur in your lifetime or eating construction dust while trying to reconstruct the shattered shreds of your life because the disaster moved faster than you did? Your choice.

Mother Nature always bats last.
Disasters happened before you were born, and they'll happen eons after you're dust. The only uncertainty is when and where the next disaster will strike.

Risk #3—Adverse Financial Cycles

Chuck Darwin was a nice guy, but grossly impractical. He focused strictly on the physical survival of the species. In a capitalistic society, economic survival is equally important. Without money, you'll soon wish you were extinct.

If you need proof that misery loves company, ponder the Great Recession we staggered through not long ago. Remember the triple whammy of falling stock prices, plummeting home values, and a dreadful economy? We watched helplessly as trillions of our hard-earned dollars flew to money heaven. Everyone from Warren Buffet to endowment fund managers got sucker punched by an incredibly deep downturn with no safe havens.

The stock market peaked in October 2007, then did a world class belly flop. In May 2011, for instance, the value of the stocks and bonds Annie B and I owned was still *far* below where they had been three-and-a-half years earlier. The stock market belatedly hit a new high in March 2013, too late for retirees who had liquidated their portfolios to survive. Not enough staying power.

The Federal Reserve Board's recession fighting policy of keeping the federal funds rate near zero drastically cut short-term interest rates. It goosed economic recovery, but caused severe collateral damage for thrifty souls who stashed cash away for retirement. Their reward was abysmally low interest rates on savings accounts and certificates of deposit (CDs).

Folks who planned to supplement their Social Security payments with interest from savings got screwed. A $250,000 nest-egg that earned $12,500 annually at 5 percent interest now yields a paltry $2,500 at 1 percent. Thrifty victims of the Fed's monetary policy are being forced to cannibalize their principal to stay alive. They're eating their seed corn. Full belly today; starve tomorrow.

Recessions are cyclical. Remember the oil crisis that brought America to its knees in the early '70s? Remember mortgage rates skyrocketing over 18 percent ten years later? Remember NASDAQ dot bombs exploding in the early 2000s? We've had two burst housing bubbles and two severe bear markets in the past twenty years. Other than stuffing a mattress with megabucks, I don't know any way you can protect yourself from periodic catastrophic fiscal carnage.

At a personal level, I offer these fiscal cautions:

Diversify, diversify, diversify. Don't put all your financial eggs in one basket—especially if the basket is equity in your home. Too many folks learned that the hard way when the real estate market tanked.

If you invest in the stock market, you'll sleep better with a diverse portfolio of boring, high-quality bonds and unexciting, well-managed mutual funds. If you're risk averse, shift more of your money from stocks into bonds as you get older to adjust for your reduced staying power. Don't overestimate the return you'll get from your portfolio.

Avoid the Bernie Madoff types who graciously offer to let you in on a "high-return, risk-free" Ponzi scheme. If it looks too good to be true, it is. Avoid deals filled with complex terms and fancy words. Good investments are straightforward and easy to understand.

Discuss your financial situation with a Certified Financial Planner. You need expert advice. I'm not an expert.

Risk #4—Accidental Death or Disability

Accidents come in two ever-popular varieties:

1. Due to no fault of your own, you're either grievously injured or killed because you had the misfortune to be in the wrong place at the wrong time.

2. Due to your very own incredible stupidity or carelessness, you indulged in some asinine act that culminated in your death or disability.

Innocent victim or had it coming? Either way, you're maimed or dead.

Vulnerability is an ambulance of many colors. It's getting hit by a drunk driver while you walk across the street in a crosswalk on a green light, fracturing your skull getting out of the shower, falling off the roof while clearing leaves

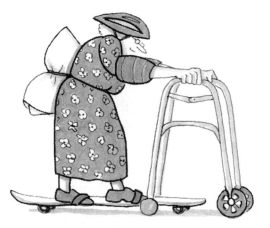

out of the rain gutter, breaking your hip falling down the stairs, or having a fatal car crash while trying to drive and talk on a cell phone.

Who amongst us *never once* changed lanes without first checking the rearview mirror and both side mirrors? Who amongst us *never once* began to cross the street before looking both ways? Who amongst us *never once* slipped in the shower? Beware. The guardian angel on our shoulder takes a day off every now and then. No point fretting about wrong place/wrong time accidents. Despite your best efforts, bad things sometimes happen to good people.

Then there are "you asked for it" dunderhead accidents. I'm pointing my finger at dunces who ignore posted warnings about riptides or thin ice. Let's not forget old fools with limited staying power who *rebuild* their houses in the middle of a flood plain or tornado corridor? Just because they survived the last disaster doesn't mean they'll be so lucky next time.

Don't be a dunderhead. No force on Earth can protect you from your own stupidity and carelessness. Until someone finds a vaccine to innoculate us against idiocy, there's no substitute for good judgment and common sense. Consider the consequences *before* you act.

Jared Diamond, author of *Guns, Germs, and Steel*, wrote an essay in the *New York Times* (January 28, 2013) about *constructive paranoia*—seeming paranoia that actually makes sense. He stressed the importance of treating low-risk hazards we encounter daily with respect. Stairs and uneven sidewalks come to mind. Unsecured area rugs, waxed floors, doorsills, shoes with slick leather soles, knives, and ladders are fraught with accident potential. I'm sure you can come up with more if you think about it. And you should.

Thanks to Mr. Diamond, I'm now a card carrying constructive paranoid about falling. You should be too. He dwelt at length on one of my favorite fears—taking a shower. Suppose the odds of injuring yourself by slipping in the shower are 1000 to 1. Not so risky, right?

Ah, but further suppose you live 16 more years and shower every day, including Feb. 29th on the four leap years? You'll have 365.25 days/year x 16 years = 5,844 opportunities to crack your skull or break a hip. If you fall only once every 1,000 showers, you can look forward to five hospital visits plus rehabs at a long-term care facility.

Unless you die. Then the other stuff is moot. Wet showers and bathtubs are slippery, hard, and super dangerous. *Always* treat them with respect. The price of carelessness is a full-body cast—or a full-body casket.

One in every three adults age 65 and older has a serious fall each year. Not boo-boos you kiss and make go away. According to the CDC, falls cause lacerations, hip/spine/hand/arm/leg/ankle or pelvis fractures, and traumatic brain injuries. We're talking about poor-Aunt-Milly-was-never-the-same-after-she-broke-her-hip falls.

Among adults 65 or older, unintentional falls are the #1 cause of injury-related death. The CDC says the first fall often leads to an even more serious fall later. For adults over 65, falls are the most common cause of nonfatal injuries and hospital admissions for trauma. From 2002 to 2012, more than two hundred thousand Americans over 65 died after a fall. Who knew?

Use handrails going up and down stairs. Install grab bars inside and outside of your tub and shower. Eliminate carpets and rugs you can trip or slip on. Watch where you're going. Failing to plan is planning to fall.

Only suckers bet against their gene pool. Only suckers bet against nature. Only suckers bet against another economic crisis. Only suckers think accidents happen just to other people. Repeat after me, "I am not a sucker."

PART TWO

DYING WELL

Chapter 6

ADVANCE DIRECTIVE

Dying well requires strategic planning abil-ity and the courage to unblinkingly confront impending rigor mortis. These aren't strong skill sets for death ostriches. Whether you're felled by a heart attack, crack your cranium in the shower, get T-boned by a red light runner, take a header off a ladder, or suffer another deadly mishap, the outcome is sadly similar. One moment you're hale and hearty; the next you're a hairy potato.

If, like me, you're a control freak, you want to direct medical decisions that affect your health care even if you're comatose. That's why you need to prepare a *written* (thanks, Sam) Advance Directive before a mishap. Unlike death ostriches, you're going to do everything you can to minimize your pain and suffering if you land in La La Land.

CHEERY FACTOID

*A verbal contract isn't worth the paper
it's written on.*
—SAM GOLDWYN

An Advance Directive (AD) has two parts:

1. **A living will** specifies the type of care and treatments you want and—equally important—don't want if you can't speak for yourself. For instance, are there baseline capabilities (walking, talking, chewing food, swallowing water safely, recognizing family and friends, etc.) you must have to make your life worth living?

   Do you, for instance, want a feeding tube permanently sewn into your stomach, so you can linger months or years in a vegetative state? If it's highly unlikely you'll ever leave La La Land, do you want electroshock zaps if your heart stops beating? How about artificial ventilation if you stop breathing? You'll find more questions to help define baseline values later in this chapter.

2. **A durable health care power of attorney (POA)** gives your health care agent—someone you literally trust with your life—the power to make health care decisions for you if you're incapacitated. Durable means your POA remains active after you're unable to speak for yourself. Your agent can be anyone at least 18 years old—your spouse or child, another relative, or someone outside your family. You also need an alternative health care agent to act on your behalf if your first choice is unavailable.

These two agents are people you trust to faithfully follow your end-of-life instructions. They must be willing and able to forcefully insist that your wishes be respected. This might mean ordering life support be discontinued if it's impossible to attain what *you* specified would be an acceptable quality of life after everything that could help you has been tried. Your agent isn't killing you—just carrying out the instructions *you* gave in your AD.

Unfortunately, there isn't a standardized AD that's accepted everywhere in America. Each state developed its own guidelines and forms. Geez! How did we get along in the good old days before dying got complicated?

You should be able to get an AD template for the state you live in from your doctor or hospital. Two online sources for your state's AD are AARP at www.aarp.org or Compassion & Choices (C&C) at www.compassionand-choices.org. C&C is the largest end-of-life-choice organization in America. Folks who aren't computer whizzes can call C&C toll free

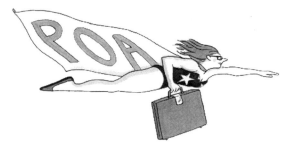

at (800) 247-7421 to get an AD and help completing it.

You don't need an attorney to complete an AD. It's legally valid after you sign it in front of the required witnesses. Disclosure: Be advised that I proudly carry membership cards in both AARP and C&C. AARP needs no introduction. It's my source for just about everything to do with aging wisely. C&C is my primary resource for info regarding end-of-life planning and choices.

C&C has a resource guide chockfull of sound advice as well as end-of-life planning ideas. For instance, it has criteria to help you select a health care agent. If you can't think of anyone to serve as your agent, C&C has an end-of-life consultation program. Their resource guide also has a section about "The Conversation"—how to discuss your wishes for end-of-life-care with your loved ones, friends, and doctor.

The resource guide can help you clarify your priorities and insure that your wishes are honored. It includes the following exciting items you probably don't know you need:

Dementia Provision: Your AD becomes operative if you're unable to make health care decisions because you're either permanently unconscious or incapacitated by a terminal illness. Ah, but what if you're suffering from Alzheimer's disease or another form of dementia, and you're neither unconscious nor terminally ill—just a zombie? That's when you'll be glad to have the dementia provision in your AD.

Values Worksheet: This is an invaluable guide for your family, friends, and health care providers if you're incapacitated. On a 0 to 4 scale, where 0 is "Not Important" and 4 is "Very Important," you rank the importance of alternatives such as

- letting nature take its course

- preserving your quality of life

- staying true to your spiritual beliefs/ traditions

- living as long as possible regardless of your quality of life

- dying quickly rather than lingering.

The Values Worksheet also has essay questions about topics such as

What will be important to you when you're dying (e.g., physical comfort, pain management, having family members present, etc.)?

How do you feel about using life-sustaining measures in the face of terminal illness? Permanent coma? Irreversible chronic illness such as Alzheimer's disease?

Do you want to know the cold, hard truth about your condition, treatment options, and chance of success for the treatments? (How can you make valid decisions about your end-of-life medical care if no one will tell you that you're dying?)

My Particular Wishes for Therapies that Could Sustain Life. Suppose your mental or physical state deteriorated precipitously, your prognosis is grave, and it's highly unlikely you'll ever be your jolly old self again. This form tells medical professionals, your health care agent, and your family how you feel about therapies to save or prolong your life. Among other things, it covers the use of antibiotics, dialysis, artificial ventilation if you stop breathing, electroshock if your heart stops beating, etc. For each option, you specify "Yes," "No," or "Trial Period" to give your doc time to see if a therapy quickly reverses your condition. If it doesn't, the doctor discontinues it.

Hospital Visitation Form: This identifies folks you want to have visiting privileges whether or not they're related to you by blood or law. It's especially important for same-sex couples who may not be formally recognized as family members.

While we're on the subject of written directives, C&C's resource guide has sections devoted to handy documents if you're eyeball-to-eyeball with death.

DNR (Do Not Resuscitate) and OOH DNR (Out-of-Hospital Do Not Resuscitate)

A DNR is a legally binding physician's order that specifically instructs health care providers not to resuscitate you. DNRs are used if you're terminally ill or extremely elderly and frail or have a medical reason why you wouldn't benefit from CPR (cardiopulmonary resuscitation) if your heart suddenly stops beating (cardiac arrest) or you suddenly stop breathing (respiratory arrest).

CPR can be a brutal procedure. It isn't always successful. Whether a DNR would be appropriate for you should be the topic of a heart-to-heart (I'm incorrigible) conversation with your doctor.

Each state has its own DNR policies and forms. Most states have laws that require hospital staff, emergency medical technicians, and paramedics to resuscitate patients in their care. A DNR order overrides state laws to resuscitate. Some states let you include DNR instructions in your AD. Others require a separate document.

If you complete a DNR order while you're hospitalized, living in a nursing home, or residing in an assisted living facility, be sure the DNR is put into your medical records. In my opinion, it's also wise to wear a DNR medallion or bracelet engraved with your DNR requirements. If you haven't guessed by now, I'm a belt and suspenders kinda guy.

Out-of-Hospital DNR (OOH DNR) orders are for terminally ill or extremely elderly and frail people who have a medical emergency at home or anywhere else outside a medical facility. Some states require that you post a brightly colored (usually vivid pink) paper copy of the OOH DNR on your refrigerator. Wearing a bracelet or medallion to indicate you have an OOH DNR makes it easier for emergency personnel to honor your wishes.

Unless otherwise instructed, emergency personnel will start life-prolonging treatments. They won't waste time searching for a DNR. It's unlikely that they'll accept a verbal DNR order. If you've decided that you want to reject all emergency resuscitation efforts, instruct your family, friends, and neighbors *not* to call 911 if they find you without a heartbeat and not breathing. More on this later in the chapter.

POLST/MOLST (Physician or Medical Orders for Life-Sustaining Treatment)

POLST/MOLST documents facilitate end-of-life medical decision making for folks with a preexisting, life-limiting condition (terminal illness, bad ticker, emphysema, etc.) or progressive frailty. If your doctor wouldn't be surprised to see you flying in formation with other angels six months to a year from now, consider executing a POLST/MOLST document.

The POLST/MOLST is a medical order. It becomes legally valid when signed by a doctor and, depending on which state you live in, either you or your legally recognized decision maker. Unlike an AD, the POLST/MOLST is brief (two to four pages max). It's a brightly colored (usually vivid pink), instantly recognizable, portable, standardized document designed for use by doctors, paramedics, police and fire departments, emergency rooms, hospitals, and nursing homes. A POLST/MOLST is sometimes used in lieu of an OOH DNR.

POLST/MOLST is meant to complement—not replace—an AD. It can, however, be used as a stand-alone document if you don't have an

AD. Check with your doctor to find out if your state has a POLST/MOLST form.

Why two different names for a document that has basically the same purpose? Turns out the document name is established by individual state law and regulatory process. Some states opted for POLST. Other states prefer MOLST. You say *po-tah-to*. I say *po-tay-to*. Whatever works.

Completing an AD doesn't guarantee your end-of-life wishes will be honored. You need to notify everyone—family, friends, physician, caregivers, health care providers, and attorneys—who may make decisions on your behalf and get buy-in from them. If everyone doesn't agree with your wishes, you're setting the stage for a mega-mess. Deathbed disputes can quickly escalate into intense emotional distress, vitriolic lawsuits, unnecessary medical expenses as well as equally unnecessary pain and suffering for you and your loved ones.

Suppose after enjoying a long, happy life filled with success and love, you end up comatose in an ICU (intensive care unit) in horrible pain with zero chance of improvement. Your exquisitely explicit AD states in that case you don't want aggressive chemo, radiation treatments, or invasive surgery that protracts your death. You only want measures to relieve pain and suffering, so you can go gently into the endless night.

Further, suppose your health care agent is fervently praying for a miraculous recovery. The agent loves you too much to let you go while there's still a single raspy breath left in your bony body. Your agent refuses to follow the instructions in your AD. Betraying your trust, the agent orders the doctor to do everything possible to prolong your miserable existence— respirators, artificial feeding, no procedure too invasive, no treatment too experimental.

Your agent prays while you suffer. Awkward.

Or it could as easily be the other way around. Suppose your AD specifies you hanker to hang around as long as humanly possible. Your agent, conversely, believes it would be cruel and unusual punishment to prolong your suffering.

We know whose wishes will prevail, don't we? Also awkward.

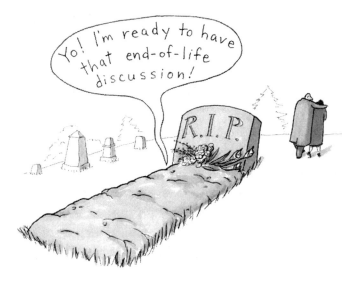

An attorney pal of mine told me a story I've never forgotten. She labored long to create a will and AD for a couple in their early 50s with teenage daughters. The couple did their best to cover every possible contingency down to and including a mutual desire to be cremated after making organ donations. They even specified precisely where they wanted their ashes scattered.

Fast forward twenty years. After a massive heart attack, the wife is in an ICU in a deep coma. Her husband and older daughter are by her side. The family doctor gently says her prognosis is hopeless. She suffered irreversible, catastrophic brain damage. There's no chance she'll have a meaningful quality of life. She'll never again be the wife and mother they know and love.

Wiping away tears, the husband tells the doc, "I'm my wife's health care agent. I know what she wants. This situation is covered in her Advance Directive. If she's in a vegetative state with no chance of recovery, she doesn't want extreme measures taken. Do not resuscitate. No ventilator or feeding tubes. Make her comfortable. Medicate her so she doesn't suffer. Let nature take its course as quickly and peacefully as possible."

The daughter interrupted, "I can't believe what I just heard, Dad. You want to murder Mother. We should do everything we can to get Mom back on her feet. As long as she's alive, there's a chance she'll recover. If you kill Mother, I'll never let you see your grandchildren again."

This hideous confrontation need not happen to you. If you discuss your end-of-life wishes with your family, your health care agent won't be forced into a ghastly choice between honoring your end-of-life wishes or acquiescing to well-intentioned emotional blackmail.

Use your Advance Directive as an end-of-life road map. You know your family dynamic better than I do. You decide whether it would be better to have one-to-one conversations with each member of your family or hold a family meeting. Either way, give everyone a copy of your AD. Go through it page by page. Spend as much time as necessary discussing your Values Worksheet and wishes regarding therapies that could sustain life.

Let everyone know whom you appointed as your health care agents and why you selected them. Tell your family you trust your agents and don't want family members to interfere with decisions they make on your behalf. (Be darn sure your agents are kindred spirits who understand and fully support your end-of-life wishes.) You might run into resistance. Some family members may not support your wishes. That's OK. People who love each other can disagree. Advise dissidents verbally (and in writing if you think it's necessary) that you don't want them to meddle with your wishes.

Your AD isn't carved in stone. Review it periodically to be sure it reflects your *current* wishes. While you're still healthy, once every five years is fine. Should you develop a life-threatening, chronic illness, more frequently is better. If you're terminally ill (six months or less to live), immediately scrutinize your AD more intensely than the IRS checks your tax return.

In a perfect world, your transition from life to death would be swift, painless, and peaceful. In the real world, who knows? That's why you must not put off The Conversation. The road to perdition is paved with good intentions. Three things are certain:

1. **There will never be an ideal time** to have an end-of-life discussion with your loved ones.

2. **The best time** to have The Conversation is before you're comatose.

3. **You can't e-mail** end-of-life instructions from La La Land.

Which brings us to the final chapter. I know you're dying to read it.

Chapter 7

A GOOD DEATH

A good death lets you control when, where, and how you die. If I were certain you'd tranquilly expire at home tenderly tucked into your comfy bed, there'd be no Chapter 7. Sadly, the odds are stacked against you.

According to Dr. Ira Byock, Director of Palliative Medicine at Dartmouth-Hitchcock Medical Center, in his book, *The Best Care Possible:*

"Nearly everyone who is asked where they would want to spend their final days says at home, surrounded by people they know and love and who love them. . . . Unfortunately, it is not the way things turn out. At present, just over one-fifth of Americans are at home when they die. Instead, over 30 percent die in nursing homes, where, according to opinion polls, virtually no one says they want to

CHEERY FACTOID

Couples who've been together a long time often die within a year of one another. Romantics attribute the caregiver's demise to a broken heart. Cynics say it's exhaustion.

be. Hospitals remain the site of over 50 percent of deaths in most parts of the country, and nearly 40 percent of people who die in a hospital spend their last days in an ICU (intensive care unit), where they will likely be sedated or have their arms tied down, so they will not pull out breathing tubes, intravenous lines, or catheters."

That *doesn't* have to be your fate. Suppose, during your battle with cancer, heart disease, or some other nemesis, your doctor recommends palliative care. Don't think, "Doc gave up. I'm a goner." You confused "palliative" care with "hospice" care. Though often used interchangeably, they have different meanings.

Palliative care (also called comfort care or supportive care) doesn't replace primary medical treatment. It's support for seriously ill people over and above curative treatment. Say you have a chronic illness. Specially trained palliative care doctors, nurses, pharmacists, social workers, therapists, spiritual advisors, and volunteers work with your other doctors to deal with your symptoms. The palliative care team focuses on managing physical, psychological, social, and spiritual needs to relieve pain and discomfort. Concurrently, they work to achieve the best possible quality of life for you and your family.

Hospice care is for terminally ill people with six months or less to live who certify they don't want more curative treatment. Hospice's goal is comfort, not cure. If your illness gets to the point where further aggressive interventions such as chemotherapy, radiation, and surgery will be more toxic then therapeutic, you need hospice. Hospice care focuses on pain management, symptom control, and getting the most out of whatever time you have left. End-of-life palliative care relieves and prevents suffering. Hospice enhances the quality of life for you and your loved ones through psychological, social, and bereavement counseling during your end-game and comforts them after you're gone.

AARP at www.aarp.org is an excellent resource for information about all aspects of palliative care and hospice. Another stellar resource is the National Hospice and Palliative Care Organization at www.nhpco.org. Ideally, the hospice you select will have palliative care consultants and an inpatient unit if your symptoms can't be managed at home. Be sure it's a Medicare-approved hospice that has at least twenty years' experience.

Don't wait till you have one foot in the grave to get hospice care. Given the advances made in pain management, gritting your teeth to stoically gut out debilitating pain is nuts. Hospice patients today have a better quality of life than John Wayne types.

Hospice may even extend your life. Read *Too Soon to Say Goodbye,* columnist Art Buchwald's memoir about his experience in the Washington Home and Hospice. Art entered hospice in February 2006, sure he'd die soon because his kidneys were shot and he didn't want dialysis. To his surprise, he thrived. Art left hospice in July 2006 and lived until January 2007. Go figure.

Dying is a crapshoot. Some deaths are short and sweet. Some folks (not you, I hope) suffer deaths emotionally and physically lacking a scintilla of control or dignity. They descend to such a profound depth of despair that they eventually dread the process of dying even more than death itself.

Sure, there are exit strategies if life becomes intolerable. You can force nature's hand by halting life-sustaining treatments such as insulin or dialysis. You can have your pacemaker turned off. You can shut your pie hole and refuse to eat or drink anything.

Terminal sedation, also called "palliative sedation," is a last resort therapy that doctors use for terminally ill patients who don't respond to pain management medications. All fluids, nutrition, and artificial life supports are withheld after sedating the patient to unconsciousness. Death due to dehydration and the patient's underlying illness or disease usually occurs five to ten days later. To avoid the appearance of euthanasia, terminal sedation's

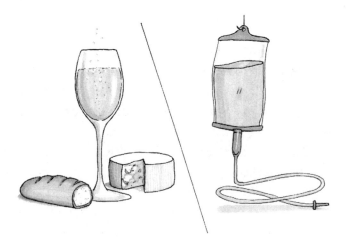

intent must be to relieve suffering, not cause death.

Geez. We wouldn't let a veterinarian put our family pet into a coma for five or ten days till it dies of dehydration. Yet we do it to human beings. What's wrong with this picture?

Dying doesn't have to be this hard. If you want more details, follow the trail I blazed for you in the Resources at the end of the book. If you'd rather cut to the chase, let's parse suicide vs. aid in dying.

When you strip out emotion, there's a clear distinction between suicide and aid in dying. Suicidal people who ultimately opt not to kill themselves go on living. That's not a choice for terminally ill people. With or without a doctor's intervention, they will die. Aid in dying allows terminally ill people to control when they die, where they die, and how much suffering they are willing to endure.

Aid in dying (also called "death with dignity") is enabling *mentally competent, terminally ill adults* to obtain a doctor's prescription for life-ending medication. Whether the patient ultimately fills the prescription is up to the individual. Some do. Others don't.

Why the nomenclature fight about "suicide" vs. "aid in dying?" Words, like stones, can wound grievously. "Surgery," for instance, is a procedure we all approach reluctantly. If it was called "stabbing," who in his right mind would have it done? Natural death advocates know "suicide" has negative connotations. They use it perniciously to forestall rational discussion.

Here's a case in point. Brittany Maynard, a 29-year-old newlywed, was diagnosed with stage 4 glioblastoma (a particularly malignant type of brain cancer) in January 2014. Brittany and her family moved from California to Oregon in June 2014, so she'd have access to Oregon's Death with Dignity Act. Brittany told *People* magazine, "For people to argue against this choice for sick people really seems evil to me. They try to mix it up with suicide, and that's really unfair, because there's not a single part of me that wants to die. But I am dying." Brittany ended her life on her terms at home on November 1st by taking the fatal dose of barbiturates prescribed by her doctor.

When I wrote this in 2016, physician aid in dying was legal in six states—Oregon (the first to legalize it), Washington, Vermont, Montana, California, and Colorado. Oregon, Washington, and Vermont laws specifically state, "Actions taken in accordance with [the Act] shall not, for any purpose, constitute suicide, assisted suicide, mercy killing, or homicide, under the law." This language was added to legally distinguish aid in dying from assisted suicide.

Death with Dignity laws vary state-to-state. In Oregon, for example, you can get a prescription for a lethal dose of barbiturates (either one hundred capsules of Nembutal or the less-expensive Seconal if you're thrifty to the end) if you satisfy these requirements:

You're a legal resident. You can't get a life-ending prescription by moving into Oregon a week before you see the black swan. Only legal residents who have relationships with local doctors qualify to obtain a prescription.

Two physicians must independently confirm you're terminally ill and only have six months or less to live. Good news (sorta). This dismal prognosis helps you qualify for hospice care under Medicare.

Two physicians must attest you're mentally competent and freely choosing aid in dying. It's natural to be depressed about dying. Doctors can distinguish between being sad because you'll never know how *House of Cards* ends and clinical depression. The doctors must counsel you about hospice and palliative pain control, attest to your absence of coercion or undue influence, and advise you that the aid in dying request is reversible.

You must make three separate requests for aid in dying. One request has to be in writing. Your two oral requests must be made at least fifteen days apart.

From what I've heard, the barbiturates taste awful. To make them more palatable, you're advised to mix the barbiturates into orange juice or some other liquid. You must drink the lethal cocktail *unassisted.* If someone helps you pour it down your throat, that's assisted suicide which is illegal in all fifty of our United States.

Approximately 32,000 Oregon residents die annually. Of the 155 Oregonians who filled the barbiturate prescription in 2014, 105 took the pills. The other 50 people died naturally, comforted by knowing they were in control of the final days of their lives. That wasn't a fluke. According to a report issued in 2015 by the Oregon Public Health Division, 1,327 terminally ill people have requested the barbiturates prescription in the seventeen years since Oregon's law took effect in 1997. Through the end of 2014, only 859 used barbiturates to end their lives.

Before deciding where you stand on aid in dying, watch Peter Richardson's documentary, *How to Die in Oregon*. You'll see terminally ill people on both sides of the issue speak for themselves. Richardson's film is heart wrenching, harrowing, inspiring, disturbing, powerful, and graphic. It's not easy to watch. I cried both times I saw it. If you're terminally ill and mentally competent, I believe you should have the right to follow *your* conscience regarding the sanctity of *your* life. If you want to hasten your end, fine. If you want to cling to every second of life no matter how dismal, also fine. Either way, it ought to be *your* choice to decide how much suffering *you* endure as your life ends.

Which brings us to end-of-life medical decisions. Nearly one-third of all Americans 65 and over had aggressive surgery in the last year of life, according to AARP's April 30, 2012, edition of *Inside E Street*. One in five had aggressive surgery in the last month of life. One in ten in the last week of life. Medicare spent $113 billion treating these patients. In many instances, this money ended up protracting death rather than extending a decent quality of life.

Most Americans face a medical system ill-suited to give us the death we want, according to the Institute of Medicine's *Dying in America* report issued in September 2014. Instead, we get breathing and feeding tubes, powerful drugs, and other treatments that often fail to extend life and can make the final days more unpleasant. The authors blame a fee-for-service medical system that offers "perverse incentives"—doctors and hospitals who end up favoring the most aggressive care, inadequate training for those caring for the dying, and physicians who default to life-saving treatment because they worry about liability.

"It's not an intentional thing. It's a systemic problem," said David Walker, former U.S. Comptroller General, who co-chaired the committee that issued the report. Doctors relentlessly seek new experimental operations, new $1,000-a-day pills, new magic to extend the spark—if not quality—of life. Sadly, most doctors aren't equally zealous about helping us die. To them, death is a failure rather than an immutable consequence of birth. What used to be one of life's most meaningful transitions is now a medical procedure.

There's a vivid distinction between extending a meaningful life and prolonging a vegetative existence defined by brain waves on a monitor and ventilator-assisted breaths per minute. Terminally ill patients deserve candid end-of-life discussions with doctors. Rather than false hope and platitudes, they need truth. You can't make good decisions without facts.

I recommend asking your doctor the following questions before you or your health care agent authorize further aggressive end-of-life interventions:

- What is the best case result if I have this intervention?

- What are my odds of success?

- What are the possible adverse repercussions? (Infection, cardiac failure, internal bleeding, paralysis, whatever—every intervention has downsides).

- What will my quality of life likely be after the intervention?

- How much longer will I live if I have the intervention?

- How much longer will I live if I opt for hospice instead of the intervention?

- Is this intervention going to extend my life or just prolong my death?

I don't know about you, but I'd happily forego a debilitating end-of-life intervention if my best-case outcome was more pain-wracked, bedridden months. I don't suffer well. Never have.

When it's my turn in the barrel, I don't want Medicare throwing money down a rat hole for end-of-life interventions that prolong my death. Wouldn't it be wonderful if the money was invested in the future by providing prenatal care for mothers, eliminating birth defects, immunizing kids against disease, and educating children so they can make the world a better place?

Just a thought.

Shortly before he died in July 1973, Dad and I were sitting in the living room of our home in Yakima, Washington, while Mom and Annie B cleaned up after dinner. Dad hardly ate a thing—just sociably pushed food around on his plate to keep us company.

I was 33 then. I'd never known anyone so close to touching death. I asked Dad how it felt to know he was dying. Dad wasn't much of a talker. He thought awhile, then ticked five points off the fingers of his left hand:

1. Cancer is no fun. I'm in a lot of pain. I don't want to die in a hospital hooked up to a machine.

2. I'm not worried about your Mother. I know you and your brothers will take care of her.

3. I'm not worried about you boys. I gave you the best gift I could. I taught you how to think.

4. I'm 74. I've had a good life. A lot of my friends have already died. It's time.

5. I'm looking forward to life's next great adventure.

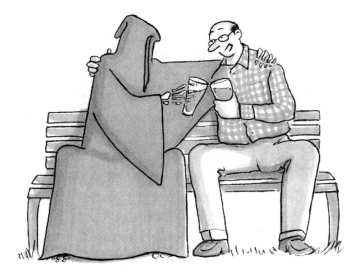

"To life!"

Two days later, after a restless night, Dad took an early morning walk. He ambled down 24th Avenue into an apple orchard two blocks from our house. Dad sat down to rest in the shade of a gnarled old apple tree close to an irrigation ditch. It was a peaceful oasis—waist-high grass waving in the summer breeze, crickets chirping, birds singing. That's where I found Dad the next afternoon. Thinking he was asleep, I shook his shoulder to wake him. I knew he'd be upset when he heard we'd been up all night looking for him.

Dad was beyond waking.

Before going home to tell Mom she didn't have to worry anymore, I communed with Dad. There wasn't a trace of pain on his face. In fact, he was smiling faintly. Other than dying on the fairway of his beloved Elks Golf and Country Club, Dad had found the perfect spot to embark on his next adventure.

We buried Dad in Seattle next to his Father. Rabbi Levine, who'd married Mom and Dad forty years earlier, officiated at Pop's funeral. After hearing how Dad looked when I found him, Rabbi Levine said he got a kiss from God. May we all be so lucky.

L'chayim. "To life" in Hebrew.

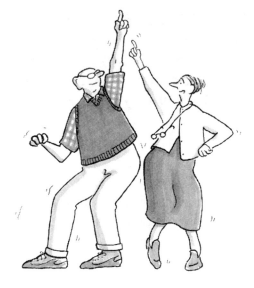

Here are some famous folks who passed on while I wrote *WTEG*. I didn't include the date each person died, but trust me, they're in chronological order. These celebrities range in age from 45 to 100. What fascinates me is how capricious Death is. He allowed some candles to burn a long time. Others he snuffed out quickly.

Richard Carlson, author of *Don't Sweat the Small Stuff,* perspired his last at 45. **George Burns**, Gracie's spouse/star of vaudeville, radio, TV, and movies, soft-shoed, cigar in hand, to 100. **Randy Pausch**, bestselling author of *The Last Lecture*, was 47 when pancreatic cancer felled him. **Roger Williams**, pianist who gained fame in 1955 with "Autumn Leaves," played to 87. **Steve Jobs**, Apple co-founder, moved to the big orchard in the sky after 56 years. **Nora Ephron**, witty screenwriter who convulsed me with "I'll have what she's having" in *When Harry Met Sally*, lay down her pen at 71. **Sally Ride**, first American women in space, was 61 when she rode into her final sunset. Her fellow astronaut, **Neil Armstrong**, first man on the moon, blasted off a month after Sally at 82. Humorist **Phyllis Diller** last cracked wise at 95. **Robin Gibb**, one of the three Bee Gees, was 62 when the disco went dark. **Peter Falk**, *Columbo* to his fans, had his series cancelled at 83. **Thomas Kinkade**, beloved by collectors and reviled by critics, painted his last cozy cottage at 54. **Stan the Man Musial**, St. Louis Cardinals baseball star, was 92 when Coach called him up to the field of dreams. **Dick Clark**, host of *American Bandstand* who shared many a New Year's Eve with us all, popped his last cork at 82. **Marvin Hamlisch**, who explained *The Way We Were* composed his farewell melody at 68. **Dr. C. Everett Koop**, four star Surgeon General, practiced what he preached to 96. **Roger Ebert**, my favorite film critic, filed his final review age 70. (Dynamic duo Siskel and Ebert became a solo act in 1999 after Death scythed Gene at 53.) Ronald Reagan's pal **Margaret Thatcher**, first female British prime minister, lived to

87. **Jean Stapleton**, Archie Bunker's sweetly naive Edith, stifled herself until 90. (**Carroll O'Connor**, Edith's oblivious bigot Archie, only blustered to 76.) The Great Hit Man nailed Tony Soprano (**James Gandolfini**) at 51. **Margaret Pellegrini**, a *Wizard of Oz* Munchkin, was 89 when she left Oz in August 2013 (only 2 of the original 124 Munchkins were still in Oz when she departed). **David Frost**, best known for interviewing Richard Nixon after Dick resigned in disgrace, was 74 when the Station Manager cut his mic. **Ray Dolby**, who took the hiss out of cassette tapes and whose sound blew us away when we saw *Star Wars*, made it to 80. **Ken Norton**, who beat Muhammad Ali in their 1973 heavyweight fight, was 70 when the Big Boxer KO'd him. Bestselling author **Tom Clancy** was 66 when he ended his *Hunt for Red October*. **M. Scott Carpenter**, second American astronaut to orbit Earth, had his final splashdown at age 88. **Nelson Mandela**, irreplaceable hero who devoted 95 years to creating justice and freedom toward a color-blind world, will be sorely missed. **Peter O'Toole**, always Lawrence of Arabia to me, was 81 when the sands of time swallowed him. Singer, songwriter **Phil Everly**,

Don's baby brother, was 74 when he last bid us *Bye Bye Love*. Ambassador **Shirley Temple Black**, most famous child movie star ever, twinkled to 85. Folk song singer and songwriter **Pete Seeger** overcame everything except death age 94. **Mickey Rooney**, America's #1 box-office draw in 1939 (the year I was born), 1940 & 1941, was 93 when his star joined the others in the sky. **Rubin "Hurricane" Carter**, middleweight boxer whose wrongful murder conviction was an international symbol of racial injustice, fought to insure justice for all until age 76. Iconically cool, impossibly handsome **Efrem Zimbalist Jr.** was 95 when he departed *77 Sunset Strip*. Crooner **Jerry Vale** was 83 when he last sang "Volare." **Maya Angelou,** civil rights activist, author, and poet sublime, graced us with her presence 86 years. **Ann B. Davis**, a.k.a. Alice Nelson, *The Brady Bunch* housekeeper, was 88 when she cleaned up her last mess. **Tony Gwynn**, San Diego Padres genius with the bat, was 54 when he headed for the field of dreams. **Louis Zamperini** was *Unbroken* for all his 97 years. Amiable **James Garner**, Bret Maverick to most of us, wisecracked his last age 86. **Lauren Bacall**, who taught Bogie how to whistle, was 89 when she took the big sleep. **Joan Rivers**, pioneering feminist comedian, laughed to 81. **Oscar de la Renta**, doyen of American fashion, designed his last wedding gown at age 82. **Ben Bradlee**, *Washington Post* editor who published the Pentagon Papers and exposed Watergate made it to 93. **Tom Magliozzi**, NPR's *Car Talk* mechanic with the infectious laugh, was 77 when he drove off. The screen darkened at 83 for **Mike Nichols**, multifaceted director of *Who's Afraid of Virginia Woolf* and *The Graduate*. **Mario Cuomo**, charismatic three-term governor of New York, termed out at 82. Pop poet **Rod McKuen** was 81 when last he rhymed. **Leonard Nimoy**, Spock to us Trekkies, was 83 when he boarded the USS *Enterprise* for his final voyage. **Jean Nidetch**, founder of Weight Watchers, kept watching till she was 91. **Frank Gifford**, the NFL great who transitioned into a *Monday Night Football* broadcasting legend, was 84 when he moved to the broadcast booth in the sky. **Julian Bond**, NAACP leader fought valiantly for civil rights and justice till he was 75. **Martin Milner**, TV star who roamed *Route 66* in a red Corvette convertible, was

83 when he ran outta gas. Bestselling author **Jackie Collins** was 77 when she lay down her pen. **Yogi Berra**, beloved baseball player, was called out at 90. Yogi once said, "Always go to other people's funerals. Otherwise they won't go to yours." Words to live by.

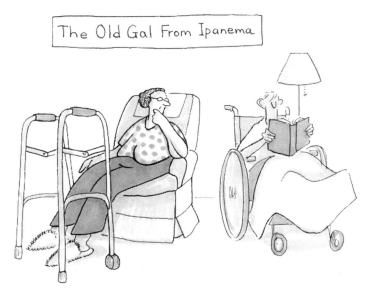

The Old Gal From Ipanema

"I was tall and tan and young and lovely.... are you listening?"

If you hanker to delve more deeply into the esoteric topic of aging gracefully and dying well, I blazed a trail for you:

Books

Art Buchwald. *Too Soon to Say Goodbye*. New York: Random House, 2006. A fine place to begin is humorist Art Buchwald's memoir about his own experiences as a hospice patient. He went into hospice expecting to kick the bucket. To his surprise and delight, he thrived. After five months in hospice, Art was discharged and lived another six months. People often live longer than expected with hospice care.

Ira Byock, M.D. *The Best Care Possible: A Physician's Quest to Transform Care Through the*

End of Life. New York: Avery, 2013. Here's a physician's perspective on hospice. Dr. Byock is one of America's foremost leaders in the field of hospice and palliative care. You'll see why he believes too many Americans suffer needlessly and die badly—and what could be done to transform end-of-life care.

Ira Byock, M.D. *Dying Well: Peace and Possibilities at the End of Life*. New York: Riverhead Books, 1998. Dr. Byock's end-of-life blueprint for dealing with doctors, how to talk to friends and relatives about life's final passage, and how to make the end of life meaningful.

Caitlin Doughty. *Smoke Gets in Your Eyes: And Other Lessons from the Crematory*. New York: W. W. Norton & Company, 2014. A fun read for the morbidly curious. Caitlin, a licensed mortician, delightfully demystifies death. Shades of the *Wizard of Oz,* Caitlin gives you a peek behind the black curtain of cremation and undertaking.

Atul Gawande, M.D. *Being Mortal: Medicine and What Matters in the End*. New York:

Metropolitan Books, 2014. You've probably seen *Being Mortal* on the bestseller list, but have you read it? After you do, you'll understand why what medicine can do often runs counter to what it should do. Surgeon Gawande will give you a wise, compassionate look at the limits of medicine in aging, frailty, and death. If you ever expect to die, read *Being Mortal*.

Nortin M. Hadler, M.D. *Rethinking Aging: Growing Old and Living Well in an Overtreated Society*. Chapel Hill: The University of North Carolina Press, 2011. Dr. Hadler looks at health care choices offered to aging Americans. He says too often these choices profit the provider rather than benefit the recipient. Rethinking Aging can help you evaluate your health care options and enable you to make informed medical choices in the last decades of your life. Dr. Hadler's pragmatic take on aging is tough love at its best.

Sherwin B. Nuland, M.D. *How We Die: Reflections of Life's Final Chapter*. New York: Alfred A Knopf, 1994. Twenty years before *Being Mortal* was published, Dr. Nuland's *How We Die* was a runaway bestseller and National Book Award winner. It is still, in my opinion, the definitive text on the varied ways death approaches us. If I could have any doctor in the world at my bedside when I die, it would be Sherwin Nuland. Another must read.

Timothy E. Quill, M.D. *Death and Dignity: Making Choices and Taking Charge*. New York: W. W. Norton & Company, 1993. In *How We Die,* Dr. Nuland called Quill's "wise and outspoken book" about a physician's role in helping mentally competent, terminally ill patients die a reference point on the compass of medical ethics. If you're concerned about unnecessary suffering and excessive aggressive medical intervention at the end of your life, this is the book for you.

Timothy E. Quill, M.D. *A Midwife Through the Dying Process: Stories of Healing & Hard Choices at the End of Life*. Baltimore: Johns Hopkins University Press, 2001. More of Dr. Quills's ideas about a better way to die. This compassionate book explores aggressive end-of-life medical intervention versus hospice-oriented care that emphasizes quality of life. In my opinion, Dr. Quill runs a close second to Dr. Nuland as the perfect doc.

Scott Taylor Smith with Michael Castleman, *When Someone Dies: The Practical Guide to the Logistics of Death*. New York: Scribner, 2013. This book will help you find your way through the quagmire of details encompassing the death of a loved one. Smith and Castleman provide checklists for everything from funeral and estate planning to navigating the complexities of online identities.

DVDs

Bill Moyers. *On Our Own Terms: Moyers on Dying*. Silver Spring, MD: Athena, 2011; original show date, 2000. If you're tired of reading, settle back in your easy chair with a big bowl of popcorn and watch Moyers's moving six-hour PBS documentary about our culture's search for "a good death." He interviews dozens of terminally ill patients as he explores the complex ethical, medical, and economic forces that shape our choices.

Peter Richardson. *How to Die in Oregon*. Corvallis, OR: Clearcut Productions, 2011. This 107-minute film won the Sundance Film Festival's 2011 Grand Jury Prize for Best Documentary. In 1994, Oregon became the first state to legalize physician-assisted death. Richardson gently enters the lives of terminally ill folks as they consider whether—and when—to end their lives by taking a lethal overdose of barbiturates. He examines both sides of what it means to die with dignity. I've watched this brilliant film twice—and wept both times.

Websites

www.aarp.org. Anyone 50 or over can join AARP. Membership in AARP doesn't make you look old. It does, however, make you a lot smarter. I've been a member for almost twenty years. AARP has become my single-best resource for info about anything and everything to do with aging gracefully and dying well.

www.compassionandchoices.org. Compassion & Choices. C&C has a much narrower focus than AARP. It's the largest end-of-life-choice organization in America. If you don't have a computer handy, you can call Compassion & Choices toll free at (800) 247-7421 for more info about death with dignity.

www.nhpco.org. National Hospice and Palliative Care Organization. NHPCO is dedicated to making hospice an integral part of America's health care system. It's a great resource for everything from education about hospice and palliative care to finding an accredited hospice in your area.

www.peninsularegent.com. The Peninsula Regent. If a picture is worth one thousand words, this website is an encyclopedia. The Peninsula Regent is my gold standard of excellence for a Continuing Care Retirement Community (CCRC). Use it as a benchmark to evaluate CCRCs in your area.

ACKNOWLEDGMENTS

Profuse thanks to Jay Schaefer, project editor; Dean Burrell, production manager and copy editor; Pamela Geismar, designer; and Julia Suits, cartoonist, who transformed my words into this book. Peter Wiley's line edits mightily smoothed the pebbles. Judy Seropan and Maura Eggan led me out of countless blind alleys. The following fabulous folks gave me insights about what worked—and what didn't: Anita Moran, Barbara Mount, Carol Kearns, Corrie Anders, Dennis Hart, Jo-Ann Rose, Dr. John Armstrong, Dr. John Fletcher, Dr. Michael Abel, Dr. Michael Turan, Dr. Robert Rodvien, Gael Bruno, Jeannine Yeomans, Joanne Wondo-lowski, Joe and Carol McLaughlin, Lynn Ogden Moore, Marc Weissman, Mary Lester, Merla Zellerbach, Nancy Lenvin, Patty Oxman, Peter and Christy Palmisano, Paula Taubman, Phil Estes, Sonja Aliesch, Trudy Drypolcher,

Valerie Crane-Dorfman, and Vince Malta. Isabelle & Serena Fritz-Cope graciously provided a quiet haven where I could write. Then there's my wonderful family—Annie B, Jeff, Jared, Genevieve, Jennifer, and Aidan—who more or less cheerfully let me ramble endlessly about the art of aging gracefully and dying well.

ABOUT THE AUTHOR

Ray Brown has been a licensed real estate broker since 1976. He coauthored two bestselling *For Dummies* books about real estate, wrote a syndicated real estate column, and hosted a call-in radio show about real estate for 16 years. Ray has spent 77 years gaining firsthand experience about aging. How well he dies is a tale yet to be told.

CPSIA information can be obtained
at www.ICGtesting.com
Printed in the USA
LVOW11s1208280317
528747LV00001B/1/P